Your Custom Roadmap for
Potentially Preventing and Curing Cancer

Reveals a Potential Method for Preventing and Curing Cancer

by
Mohan Doss, PhD

First Edition
Version 1.06
July 21, 2020

ISBN: 9781710663839
Publisher: Mohan Doss
Copyright © 2020 by Mohan Doss

For permissions please contact the author at: i4r@mail.com

Supplementary material related to this book can be accessed at the book website: https://bit.ly/2E1JHxj

Book Cover artwork designed by Katie Solkov.

CONTENTS

DISCLAIMERS

This book presents the author's views on the reasons for the development of cancer, its prevention, and treatment based on an analysis of the scientific literature. These are for your information only and are not medical advice. The reader may utilize the ideas presented in the book only after consultation with and under the supervision of a qualified health-care professional.

The views presented in this book are the author's professional opinions and do not necessarily represent the views of his employer or the organizations he is affiliated with.

LIST OF TABLES

LIST OF FIGURES

ACKNOWLEDGMENTS

First of all, I would like to thank Drs. Rosaleen Parsons and Michael Yu for their encouragement and support of my work over many years without which this book would not have been possible.

Since the book is aimed at a general audience in addition to the professionals in the field of cancer, I obtained feedback for drafts of the book from those who are not working in the cancer field in addition to those working in it. The feedbacks have led to many major improvements in the book, and so I am very grateful to all the reviewers of the drafts of the book. As I took the final decision on the contents of the book, the errors and omissions in the book should be attributed to me alone.

Among the colleagues who provided very valuable feedback include Drs. Rosaleen Parsons, Michael Yu, R. Katherine Alpaugh, and Paul F. Engstrom.

Several of my colleagues who are members of the group Scientists for Accurate Radiation Information (SARI), gave me important ideas and comments. These include Mr. Charles Pennington, Drs. Bill Sacks, James Welsh, and Yehoshua Socol.

I also wish to acknowledge the very helpful comments from my sons Jayanth and Prashanth, my brother Kantesh, and his wife Komala. In addition, I wish to thank my son Prashanth and his wife Jackie for help with the book cover and Katie Solkov for designing the artwork on the book cover.

- Mohan Doss

PREFACE

This book has been written for the general public as well as professionals who are interested in preventing and curing cancer. I have tried to use language that would be understandable by the lay person and have cited references to discuss and justify the concepts presented. I am hopeful that professionals in the field would find the information in the book helpful for improving the care of cancer patients, identifying promising avenues of research, and/or for guiding the public on the prevention of cancer. I am also hopeful that members of the public would find the information in the book helpful in establishing a custom roadmap for potentially preventing and curing cancer, in consultation with their qualified health-care professionals.

Have you or any of your loved ones been diagnosed with cancer and undergone treatments with adverse side effects? Have you wished there were effective cancer treatments with few or no adverse side effects? Have you or your loved ones wished there were ways of avoiding cancer and the pain and suffering associated with it? Have you or your loved ones worried about the false positive results from cancer screening? Have any of your loved ones died from cancer and you wished there was an effective cure for cancer? Have you been frustrated by the limited progress in preventing cancer in spite of the tremendous public expenditures in the field over the years? Have you or any of your loved ones been diagnosed with cancer and are not satisfied with the recommended watchful waiting approach? If the answer is yes to one or more of such questions, you may find some helpful answers in this book, since the book is the result of my search for answers to such questions.

You may wonder what my background is, and why I am writing a book on this subject. I am a medical physicist providing physics support for diagnostic imaging techniques such as positron emission tomography (PET) and computed tomography (CT) which involve the exposure of patients to ionizing radiation. Some years ago, when publications made claims that CT scans could cause cancers, I took the finger-pointing seriously and investigated the topic thoroughly by examining the relevant publications. **What I found was that the claims were completely without merit and, in fact, there was considerable reasoning and evidence to indicate that small amounts of radiation, equivalent to that from several CT scans, could reduce the risk of cancers.**

As I studied the subject further, I came to realize that the development of cancer (uncontrolled multiplication of cells) is not primarily due to genetic mutations, as is commonly assumed. As evidence, almost everyone has cancerous or pre-cancerous cells in their bodies but everyone does not have cancer. When I came to know of the tremendously increased cancer risk in patients whose immune system is suppressed, for example, organ-transplant recipients and AIDS patients, I realized that the immune system plays an extremely important role in preventing cancers. This led me to propose the hypothesis that the development of clinical cancer, i.e., uncontrolled multiplication of cells, is primarily caused by the weakening or suppression of the immune system. I found that there is plenty of evidence to support this hypothesis. With this hypothesis, it becomes obvious how we can approach the prevention and treatment of cancer.

Since, the weakening or suppression of the immune system may be the most important factor contributing to the development of cancer, we should be able to prevent and treat most cancers by boosting the immune system. There are indeed many methods (interventions) to boost the immune system. It occurred to me that if we enhanced the immune system with many different interventions, multiple components of the immune system would be boosted so that none of them would be weak, thereby making it harder for the cancer cells to overcome the immune system. However, all the interventions would not be applicable or acceptable to everyone, and so we should let the individuals choose which interventions they would like to use. This led me to propose "Individualized Interventions to Improve the Immune Response (I^4R)" (pronunciation key: eye-four-ahr) as an approach to treat cancer.

One advantage of this approach is that there would be few adverse side effects from the interventions. Therefore, the approach would be welcomed by cancer patients and their loved ones. Another point to be noted is that many immune boosting interventions are already known to have a cancer preventive and/or therapeutic effect. A third advantage is that many of the interventions would improve health in other ways, in addition to reducing cancer. These and other advantages of the I^4R approach indicate that the method holds great promise for dealing with cancer. Hence, I decided to write this book and share the excitement with the general public and the professionals. Of course, a considerable amount of research including clinical trials needs to be conducted to determine the effectiveness of this approach.

The current standard of care for cancer patients does work well for some cancer patients, but for others, the results have not been good, because the treatments are ineffective or become ineffective after a period of time. In addition, the adverse side effects of the treatments can reduce the quality of life. Notwithstanding these issues, the benefits of the current treatments have been well established, and patient outcomes have been worse when they have refused the traditional treatments. **Therefore, the current standard of care should continue to be used for cancer patients while exploring any new proposed approaches through pilot clinical trials.**

If the pilot clinical trials demonstrate that a new approach is effective in treating cancer, more detailed clinical trials would need to be conducted. If these clinical trials also demonstrate the effectiveness of the new approach and if its performance is better than the traditional approach, the medical community would be justified in adopting the new approach. Since the entire process of validating the new approach would take a considerable amount of time to accomplish, it is important to start the pilot clinical trials promptly. **Until the detailed clinical trials are completed, the results are satisfactory, and the medical community adopts the new approach, the current approach should continue to be used for treating cancer patients.**

Because of this situation, that the approach I have suggested has not been validated in clinical trials, this book should be considered as a work in progress. This is the reason for the adverb "potentially" in the title of the book. The clinical trials would show what fraction of cancers are effectively prevented and treated by the I^4R approach. Optimistically, the approach would be successful in preventing and treating all the cancers. It is quite possible that some cancers would not be prevented or treated effectively by the approach, and for such cancers, the traditional treatments would be needed. I plan to publish updates to the book when the results of the clinical trials become available. I also plan to update the book periodically based on the feedback obtained from the readers. Self-publishing the book makes it more convenient to publish such updates.

The approach to cancer prevention and treatment presented in this book, if it is studied, validated in clinical trials, and adopted, may be helpful in preventing the development of cancer, and in case cancer develops, may be helpful in treating it effectively with very few adverse side effects, thereby revolutionizing the cancer field.

INTRODUCTION

Chapter 1 provides some background information on the results from the present approach to cancer, and explains why a better approach is needed.

Chapter 2 discusses what the primary reason for the development of cancer (uncontrolled multiplication of cells) is. It begins with the discussion of the tremendous increase in the cancer rates when the immune system is suppressed, and hypothesizes that weakening or suppression of the immune system may be the primary reason for the development of most cancers. Then it presents a considerable amount of evidence to support the hypothesis. Based on this hypothesis, we should be able to prevent and treat most cancers by boosting the immune system.

Chapter 3 gives a brief discussion of the immune system, discusses many interventions that would boost the immune system, and notes that different interventions may activate different components of the immune system, and some components of the immune system may not be activated by some of the interventions.

Chapter 4 introduces the hypothesis that when the efficiencies of some immune system components decline below certain critical levels, cancer could develop. Based on this concept, cancer could be prevented or treated by boosting the efficiencies of these critical components. Since a single intervention may not boost the critical components of the immune system, using multiple interventions may be important to improve the likelihood that the critical components are boosted. However, all the immune-boosting interventions would not be applicable or acceptable to everyone, and so the choice of the interventions needs to be individualized. This approach, called "Individualized Interventions to Improve the Immune Response (I^4R)" (pronunciation key: eye-four-ahr), needs to be studied in clinical trials to determine if it is successful in preventing and treating cancer.

Chapter 5 compares the I⁴R approach with the current approach to cancer and explains that it may overcome many of the disadvantages of the present approach.

Chapter 6 estimates the likely effectiveness of the I⁴R approach for preventing and treating cancer. Since substantial reductions of cancer incidence and mortality rates have been observed with many of the individual immune boosting interventions, it is possible that multiple interventions could result in even larger reductions in the cancer incidence and mortality rates than those observed with the individual interventions.

Chapter 7 discusses the actions that need to be taken to facilitate the clinical trials of the I⁴R approach. Many of the immune boosting interventions are lifestyle interventions, which are harder to achieve on a consistent basis. Therefore, it is essential that we study all the possible non-lifestyle-based interventions. However, there are major hurdles for studying one such intervention, low-level radiation, and the hurdles need to be overcome in order to be able to study the intervention in clinical trials. It then describes the clinical trials that can be conducted to determine the usefulness of the I⁴R approach for cancer prevention, treatment, and screening. It points out that it is important to conduct the clinical trials promptly to validate the I⁴R approach.

Chapter 8 presents my pitch explaining why you, the reader, should support the clinical trials of the I⁴R approach to cancer, and suggests ways in which you can help.

Appendix A discusses how we can enable the study of low-level radiation as an intervention to boost the immune system.

Appendix B provides brief primers on the two opposing models for the effect of low-level radiation on cancer, radiation hormesis and the linear no-threshold (LNT) model.

Appendix C gives answers to some frequently asked questions regarding the book and its contents.

1. BACKGROUND

Cancer is the most feared disease in the western world [1]. USA declared a war on cancer in the 1970s [2], and considerable resources have been devoted to cancer research since then both in the USA and worldwide [3]. A vast amount of knowledge has been accumulated about the nature of cancer, hallmarks of cancer have been identified [4-5], and many advances have taken place in the areas of cancer screening, diagnosis, and treatment [6-7]. However, there are indications that we are far from winning the war on cancer [8-9].

Progress in the War on Cancer

Let us examine how the cancer mortality rate has changed in the USA in the recent years. Figure 1 shows the age-adjusted mortality rates for cancer and heart disease in the USA for the past five decades [10].

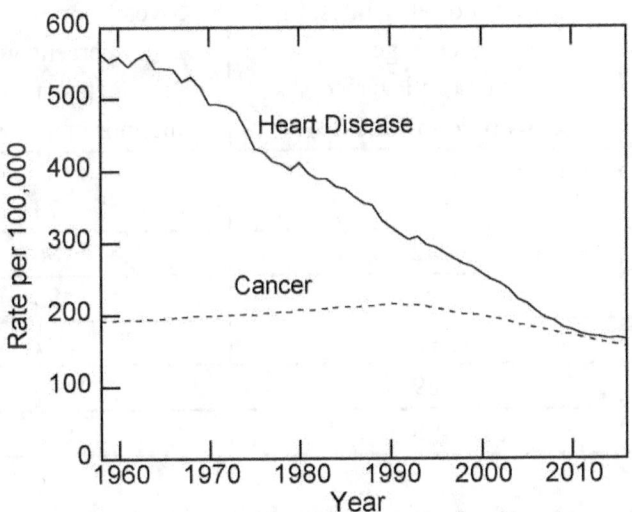

Figure 1. Age-adjusted mortality rates for heart disease and cancer in the USA for 1958-2016 [10]. Note: Age-adjusted mortality rate is a calculated mortality rate that accounts for the age distribution of the population.

Whereas there has been a major decline in the age-adjusted mortality rate for heart disease during the past five decades, the rate for cancer has declined only modestly. In fact, cancer is predicted to become the leading cause of death in the USA overtaking heart disease in the near future [11].

Now let us examine how we have progressed in treating metastatic cancer, i.e. cancer that has spread from its initial location to another part or other parts of the body. Table 1 compares the 5-year mortality rates for patients with metastatic cancer diagnosed in 1986-1993 with those diagnosed two decades later, for the top six deadliest cancers.

Table 1. Comparison of the 5-year mortality rates of metastatic cancer patients diagnosed during 1986-1993 and 2008-2014, for the top six deadliest cancers. The data are derived from the American Cancer Society's Cancer Facts and Figures Reports for the years 1998 and 2019.

Cancer Type	5-year mortality rates, in percentages, for metastatic cancers diagnosed in 1986-1993	5-year mortality rates, in percentages, for metastatic cancers diagnosed in 2008-2014
Breast (female)	79	73
Colon	92	86
Lung	98	95
Pancreas	98	97
Prostate	69	70
Rectum	95	85

There has been only a modest reduction in the 5-year mortality rates for these metastatic cancers over the two decades.

Future Outlook for the War on Cancer

In a recent interview, the Co-Chair of the President's Council of Advisors on Science and Technology stated that it may take another 30 or 40 years to cure the majority of cancers or even convert them into completely treatable, manageable diseases. He also said that 'cure' for most or all cancer types in the next few years "is not a promise we can deliver". A survey of a large number of professionals working in the cancer field has indicated that a majority of the respondents do not expect a cure for cancer to be discovered in the near future [12]. This situation is quite unsatisfactory for cancer patients and the public. It is clear that a better approach to cancer is needed [9]. In this book, I have presented what I consider to be a better approach to cancer.

In my view, the main reason the war on cancer appears to have faltered is that there has been a major misunderstanding of the primary reason for the development of cancer. What is the primary reason for the development of cancer? That will be the subject of the next chapter.

2. THE PRIMARY REASON FOR THE DEVELOPMENT OF CANCER

In order to win the war on cancer, the most important question that needs to be answered correctly is "What is the primary reason for the development of cancer?" If we do not answer this question correctly, our efforts will not bear much fruit, however many resources we devote to the problem and however hard we try. For example, if we try to solve the problem of high fever by using many different methods of cooling the body such as icepacks, cold showers, etc., the relief, if any, would be temporary. Whatever methods we use and however much resources we devote to reducing the body temperature in this manner would not solve the problem of high fever. Instead, if we identify the reason for the development of high fever as an infection, and deal with the infection with antibiotics, assuming our body is not able to deal with the infection on its own, the problem of high fever would be solved. When we attack a major problem with large amounts of efforts and resources but do not make much progress, it may indicate that we may not be addressing the primary reason for the problem. This may be the explanation for the present situation with respect to the war on cancer, where real progress has been painfully slow and no solution is in sight, in spite of tremendous expenditures and the large number of reported advances in the field.

Is Cancer a Genetic Disease?

It is commonly assumed that cancer is a genetic disease caused by genetic mutations in cells that make the cells divide uncontrollably, giving rise to cancer. This concept of cancer is known as the mutation model of cancer [13]. Cancer cells can develop through random errors occurring in the DNA due to natural causes within the cells [14]. They can also develop due to external causes like smoking [15].

The current predominant view is that cancer is the result of the gradual accumulation of driver gene mutations (driver gene mutations = mutations that help increase the growth rates of cells) [14]. However, recent investigations have shown that there is a considerable occurrence of driver gene mutations in the normal cells of individuals who have not been diagnosed with cancer [16-17], indicating that driver gene mutations may not necessarily imply cancer.

There is plenty of evidence indicating that increased mutations do not imply increased cancers. Accumulated mutations in the spleen of mice increase the most during the young age but lymphoma, a type of cancer, occurs at the lowest rate during the young age (Figure 2) [18], indicating that an increase in the mutations does not necessarily imply increased cancers.

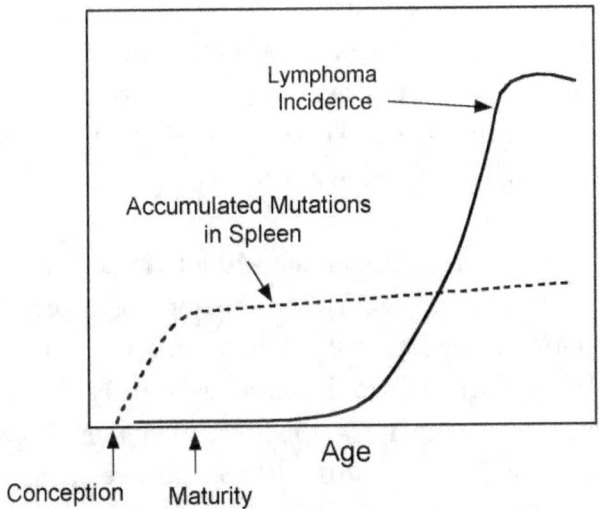

Figure 2. Schematic depiction of accumulated mutations in spleen of mice and lymphoma incidence as a function of age. Data from [18].

For humans, children have the lowest cancer rates [19] though they would be accumulating mutations at the highest rates. DNA repair deficiency is noted in the disease conditions known as Cockayne's syndrome and trichothiodystrophy but increased cancer risk is not observed for patients with these conditions [20]. Autopsy studies have shown the presence of cancer cells corresponding to various cancers, e.g., prostate [21], breast [22], renal cell carcinoma [23], and pancreatic cancer [24], in the bodies of patients but the patients were not diagnosed with the cancers. All these data indicate that increase in the mutations or the formation of cancer cells does not necessarily imply real cancers.

Whereas almost everyone may have covert cancers (cancer cells or pre-cancerous cells) in their bodies [25] everyone does not have cancer. Even among newborns, one in twenty have pre-leukemic cells (a precursor to leukemias) but childhood leukemia rates are 100 times lower, indicating that pre-leukemic cells in most of the newborns do not become real leukemias during their childhood [26]. Why is it that in the vast majority of the children, pre-leukemic cells do not develop into real leukemias, and why is it that in most of us, the presence of cancerous or pre-cancerous cells does not imply cancer? **The main reason is the immune system, since it is able to eliminate the cancer cells [27] or keep them under control preventing them from multiplying and growing into a tumor [28]. We really have to thank our immune system for keeping us safe from cancer.**

Immune Suppression Model of Cancer

Since the immune system plays a major role in keeping the cancer cells under control, if the immune system is weakened or suppressed, we can expect the cancer risk to increase drastically. This was indeed observed in the study of organ-transplant recipients (in whom the immune system is suppressed) in the 1970s [29] and has been confirmed in more recent studies [30-31]. For young organ-transplant recipients, cancer mortality rate increases by a factor of about 50 (Figure 3) [32], which is a huge increase indeed.

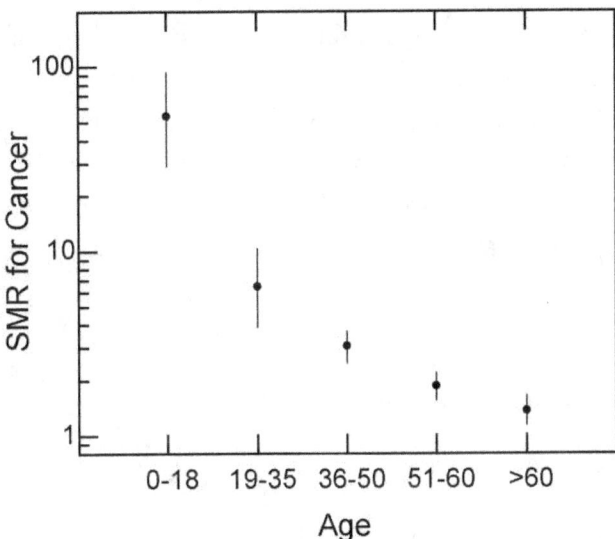

Figure 3. Standardized mortality ratio (SMR) for cancer in organ-transplant recipients as a function of age. Data from [32]. SMR is the ratio of the number of observed deaths to the number of expected deaths.

Patients with acquired immunodeficiency syndrome (AIDS), in whom the immune system is suppressed, also have an increased risk of cancer [33]. Children with AIDS face a 40-fold increase in cancer risk [34], which is again a huge increase. Such a large increase in the cancer risk when the immune system is suppressed indicates that the immune system plays a very important role in preventing cancers. Therefore, when mutations accumulate due to internal or external causes, cancer cells may form, but the immune system may eliminate them. Another possibility is that when cancer cells form, the immune system is not able to eliminate them completely but it is able to keep them in check, i.e. it is able to prevent them from multiplying out of control, resulting in covert cancers. In this phase, known as the equilibrium phase, mutations may develop among the cancer cells that enable them to hide from the immune system, and those cancer cells would be able to multiply unchecked, in spite of the immune system, resulting in immune system evading cancers [35].

Another way in which cancer could develop is when the immune system capacity weakens. When the immune system becomes weak or is suppressed, covert cancers, or any new cancer cells that are formed, would be able to multiply uncontrollably causing real cancer. I refer to this concept as the immune suppression model of cancer [36]. Let us see if the immune suppression model of cancer is able to explain qualitatively the well-known increase in the cancer mortality rate with age (Figure 4).

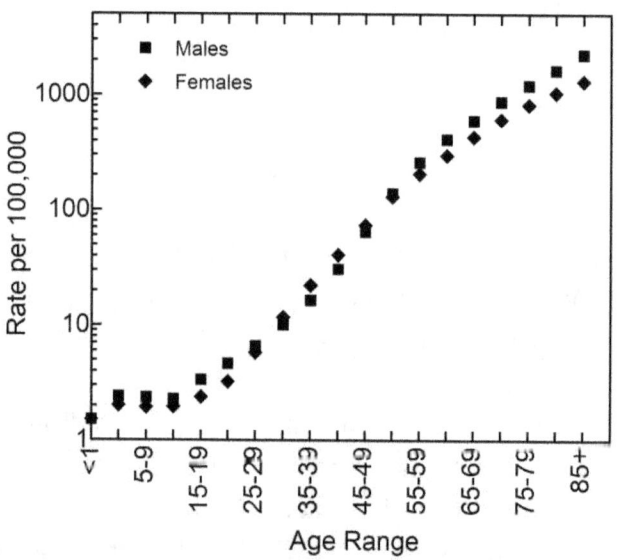

Figure 4. Annual cancer mortality rate in the USA as a function of age for 2012-2016. Data from NCI's SEER Explorer.

Since many immune system components decline with age, e.g., thymus gland [37], natural killer cells [38], and white blood cells [39]), and the immune system response declines rapidly with age (Figure 5) [40], based on the immune suppression model of cancer, cancer risk would increase with age, providing a qualitative explanation for the age dependence of the cancer mortality rate.

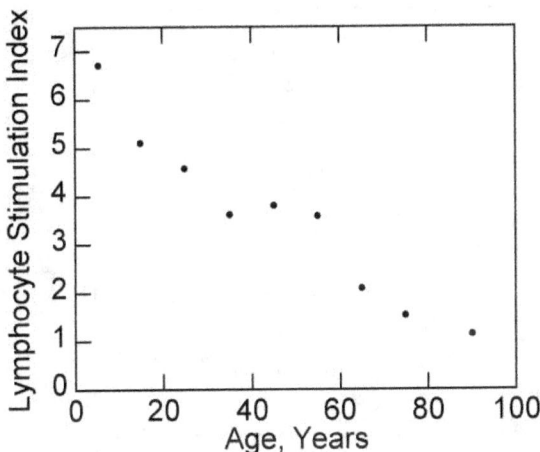

Figure 5. Lymphocyte stimulation index (an indicator of immune system response to vaccination) as a function of age. Data from [40].

An analysis has shown that the age dependence of many types of cancers can be explained using the immune suppression model of cancer [41] (Note: the publication refers to it as the immunological model of cancer), providing an alternative to the explanation traditionally provided using the mutation model of cancer [13,42].

The occurrence of almost all cancers increases with age, and this is generally explained using the mutation model of cancer because mutations increase with age. However, for a couple of situations, cancer risk decreases with age, and these would be difficult to explain using the mutation model of cancer.

As an example, the incidence of testicular cancer is known to decrease with age, for ages>30 (Figure 6).

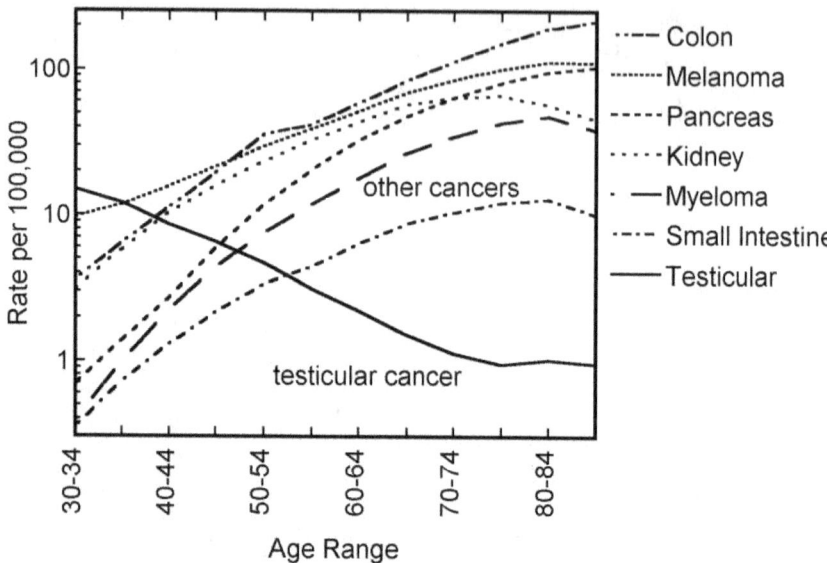

Figure 6. Cancer incidence rate as a function of age for testicular cancer compared with a few types of cancers in the USA during 2012-2016, for ages>30. Data from SEER Explorer.

The mutation model of cancer cannot explain the decrease in the incidence of testicular cancer with age whereas there is a qualitative explanation using the immune suppression model of cancer.

At puberty, when the production of sperm begins, the immune system within the testes is suppressed in order to protect the sperm [43]. Fertility of males peaks at about 30 years of age [44] when the immune system would be suppressed the most in the testes. Based on the immune suppression model of cancer, we would expect the cancer risk in the testes to peak at this age, and this has indeed been observed [45]. For ages greater than 30, fertility of males declines steadily with age [44]. Therefore, there would be reduced suppression of the immune system with age (i.e. enhancement of the immune system with age) in the testes and so the testicular cancer risk would decrease with age, based on the immune suppression model of cancer.

Another puzzling aspect of the age dependence of cancer is that cancer mortality rate decreases with increasing age for ages greater than 85 [46]. This aspect of cancer mortality rate also would not be explicable with the mutation model of cancer whereas there is a qualitative explanation using the immune suppression model of cancer.

It has been observed that among the people aged 80 and over, those with the lowest immune response had 80% all-cause mortality rate within two years whereas those with higher immune response had 35% all-cause mortality rate within the same period [47]. The increased deaths in the people with the lowest immune response implies that the survivors would have, on the average, increased immune response in comparison to the population a few years earlier. Therefore, based on the immune suppression model of cancer, cancer mortality rate would be expected to decrease as age increases above 85.

Though these are qualitative explanations for the two observations, even qualitative explanations would be difficult based on the mutation model of cancer. Now let us discuss the available evidence for the immune suppression model of cancer.

Evidence to Support the Immune Suppression Model of Cancer

There is a considerable amount of evidence to support the immune suppression model of cancer, in the form of increased cancers when the immune system is weakened or suppressed and decreased cancers when the immune system is enhanced (Table 2).

Table 2. Observed negative correlation between the change in the immune system response and the cancer rates, i.e. when the immune system response increases, cancer rate decreases, and vice versa. Note: ↑ indicates increase, and ↓ indicates decrease.

Aspect	Change in immune response	Observed effect on cancer rate
Prolonged sitting (Inactivity)	↓ [48]	↑ [49]
Cigarette smoking	↓ [50]	↑ [50]
Alcohol abuse	↓ [51]	↑ [52]
Light at night	↓ [53]	↑breast cancer risk [54]

Circadian disruption (disturbance of the 24-hour sleep-wake cycle)	↓ [55]	↑breast cancer risk [56]
Surgery	↓ [57]	↑ [58]
Ulcerative colitis, chronic pancreatitis, gastritis, chronic hepatitis (inflammation of the colon, pancreas, stomach lining, and liver, respectively), and lung inflammation	↓ [59]	↑colorectal cancer [60], pancreatic cancer [61], gastric cancer (cancer in the lining of the stomach) [62], hepatocellular carcinoma (cancer of the liver) [63], and mesothelioma (cancer in the tissue surrounding the lungs) [64]
Xeroderma pigmentosum (a very rare skin disorder where a person is highly sensitive to sunlight)	↓ [20]	↑skin cancer [20]
Children with Down's syndrome	↓ [65]	↑childhood cancers [66]
Maternal alcohol abuse	↓ [67] (increased neonatal infections)	↑infant leukemias [67]
Obstructive sleep apnea (blockage of upper airway while sleeping)	↓ [68]	↑cancer incidence [69]
Exposure to high-level radiation	↓ [70]	↑ [71]
Allergy sufferers	↑Immunoglobulin E [72]	↓cancer risk [73]
Exercise	↑ [74]	↓cancer mortality rate [75]
Infections	↑ [76]	↓ [77]
Childcare attendance	↑due to frequent infections [78]	↓childhood leukemias [79]
Flu vaccination	↑ [80]	↓cancer mortality rate [81]

Weight loss following bariatric (weight reduction) surgery	↑ [82]	↓ [83]
Exposure to low-level radiation	↑ [84]	↓ [85]
Breastfeeding (effect on child)	↑ (in infants) [86]	↓childhood leukemias [87]

The large negative correlation noted above between the immune system response and cancer risk indicates that most cancers may develop due to the weakening or suppression of the immune system, and not due to the immune system evading cancers. Another way of interpreting this observation is that the boosted immune system may be able to overcome the immune system evasion, if any, by the cancer cells.

How can we confirm that the suppressed immune system results in increased incidence of cancer? In a study conducted in Japan, the ability of white blood cells to destroy cancer cells was measured as an indicator of immune response in 3,625 men and women greater than 40 years of age, and they were followed up for about 11 years to determine their cancer rates. People whose immune system responses were at a low level were found to have much higher cancer rates during the subsequent 11 years when compared to the cancer rates in the people whose immune system responses were at medium or high levels (Figure 7) [88].

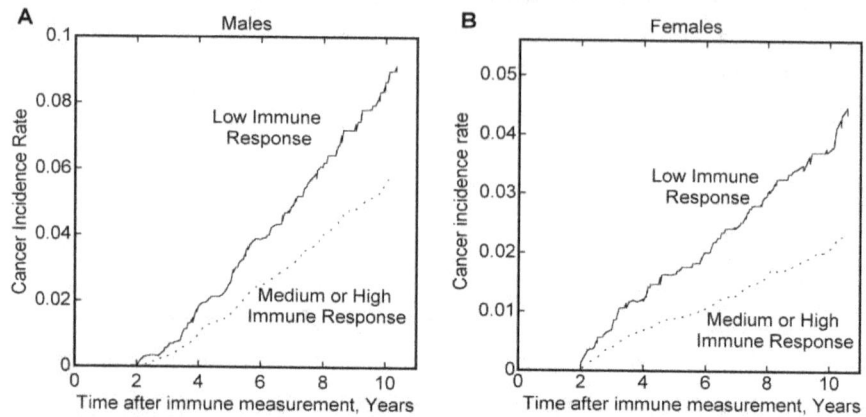

Figure 7. Cumulative cancer incidence rates for (A) Males and (B) Females in the years after the measurement of the immune response, for those with low immune response and those with medium or high responses. Cancers in the first two years after the measurement of the immune response were not considered in the study, to reduce the possibility that an existing cancer may have affected the immune system response measurement. Data from [88].

These data provide strong support for the concept that a weak immune system increases cancer risk, consistent with the immune suppression model of cancer.

For breast cancer patients also, a similar observation has been made. In a study of early-stage breast cancer patients, those with the higher functioning of the natural killer cells (a type of white blood cells) had reduced recurrence of breast cancer [89].

In summary, though mutations are necessary for the development of cancer, they are not sufficient because the immune system can eliminate the cancer cells or keep them under control. The observed large negative correlation between the immune system response and cancer risk supports the hypothesis that the primary reason for the development of cancer is the weakening or suppression of the immune system, which enables cancer to grow.

Based on this concept, we should be able to reduce the cancer incidence and mortality by improving the immune response. How can we improve the response of the immune system? That is the subject of the next chapter.

3. INTERVENTIONS TO IMPROVE THE IMMUNE SYSTEM RESPONSE

The immune system protects us from external hazards such as harmful bacteria and viruses that may enter our body as well as internal hazards such as tumor cells [90]. The immune system is very complex with many different components. Some components of the immune system move in the body through blood and lymph fluid while others reside in the various tissues and organs. Some components of the immune system detect foreign objects and tumor cells. Others send signals when the offenders are detected. There are also components that attack the offenders to destroy them. There are many more components with additional roles to play. Some of the immune system components perform multiple functions, and there is a considerable amount of redundancy built into the immune system, as several different components perform the same or similar functions. Due to such redundancies built into the immune system and the excess capacity of the components, the immune system, when it is functioning properly, is extremely effective in neutralizing the external and internal hazards we may face. Considering that so many different components are involved in the functioning of the immune system, how can we improve the immune system response, i.e., the effectiveness of the immune system in eliminating the foreign invaders and cancer cells? We can do this by improving the performance of one or more components of the immune system.

Interventions to Improve the Immune System Response

There are several actions that one can take to improve the immune system response. I am referring to these as interventions. Many publications have reported on the performance of the various components of the immune system following the interventions, and I have compiled some of them in Table 3.

Table 3. The effects of the immune system boosting interventions on some components or aspects of the immune system. Some of the immune system components that were observed to be enhanced (or the observed effects of the immune system enhancement) are listed in the second column. The third column shows the components that were not enhanced following the interventions. Note: ↑ indicates increase, ↓ indicates decrease, and → indicates no change.

Note: I have shown the technical terms for the immune system components or the immune system enhancements, in order to bring to your attention the observation that different components of the immune system have been stimulated by different interventions. Understanding the meanings of these technical terms is not needed for the subsequent discussion, and so these technical terms are not explained here.

Immune system boosting intervention	Some of the observed effects of the immune system enhancement	Aspects of the immune system that were not enhanced
Physical activity or exercise [91]	↑Mobilization of NK cell, T cell, and B cell	
Dance [92]	↑IL-2 levels	
Physical activity in elderly women [93]	↑NK-cell cytotoxicity, T-cell proliferation	→Lymphocyte counts
Endurance training in elderly men [94]	↑IL-2, IL-4 and IFN-γ production, T-cell proliferation	→NK-cell cytotoxicity, Lymphocyte counts
Daily exercise in elderly men [95]	↑Neutrophil phagocytosis	→NK-cell activity
Aerobic exercise in elderly men and women [96]	↑T-cell proliferation, NK-cell cytotoxicity	→Neutrophil, lymphocyte, CD4+ and CD8+ T-cells, monocytes
Exercise in breast cancer survivors [97]	↑Unstimulated T-cell proliferation, NK-cell cytotoxicity	→neutrophil oxidative burst, T-cell, B-cell, NK-cell numbers

Moderate exercise in the elderly [98]	↑Response to flu vaccination	
Sauna [99]	↑White blood cells, lymphocyte, neutrophil and basophil counts	
Cold shower [100]	↑leukocytes, neutrophil percentage	→ Inflammation markers IL-6, TNF-α
Forest bathing trips (leisurely trips to the wilderness) [101]	↑NK-cell activity	
Living at a high elevation [102]	↑NK cells, White blood cells, B-cells	
Sunlight exposure [103]	↑T-cell function	
Yoga [104]	↑IL-12 and IFN-γ	→Inflammation marker TNF-α
Rhythmic breathing [105]	↑Number of NK cells	
Meditation [106]	↓Inflammation marker: CRP; ↑telomerase activity,	→ IL-1, IL-6, IL-8, IL-10, IFN-γ, Inflammation marker TNF-α
Laughter [107]	↑NK-cell activity	
Tai chi [108]	↑Ratio of CD4:CD8 cells, CD4CD25 regulatory T cells	→Total white blood cell count, CD4 and CD8 counts
Acupuncture [109]	↑NK-cell activation, IL-2, IFN-γ, SPI1 pathway	
Smoking cessation [110]	↑NK-cell cytotoxic activity	→lymphocyte proliferation
Calorie restriction (30% reduction of food intake) in overweight adults [111]	↑Delayed-type hypersensitivity, T-cell proliferation	

Calorie restriction [112]	↓Inflammation markers: CRP, leptin, TNF-α, and ICAM-1	
Intermittent fasting [113]	↓Inflammation markers TNF-α, IL-1β, IL-6	
Fruit-vegetable consumption [114]	↑NK-cell numbers, NK-cell cytotoxicity, Response to Pneumovax II vaccination	→Response to tetanus vaccination
Vitamin D supplementation (if deficient) [115]	↓infections	
Yogurt [116]	↑IgA secreting cells	→IgG secreting cells, CD4+ T-Cells
Probiotic foods [117]	↑Phagocytosis, NK-cell activity, antibody response to immunization	
Whole grains [118]	↑Effector memory T cells	→IFN-γ, IL-10, IL-6, IL-8, IL-1β
Consumption of deuterium-depleted water [119]	↑Polymorphonuclear leukocytes (PMNs), lymphocytes, Phagocytic capacity of PMNs	
Low-dose aspirin [120]	↓Inflammation	
Statins [121]	↑Activation of NK cells	
Avoid excessive alcohol consumption [51]	↑NK-cell cytotoxicity, function of dendritic cells, monocytes, macrophages, IFN-γ, T-cell response, CD8+ T Cells, B cells; ↓Pro-inflammatory cytokine TNF-α	
Reduce red meat in diet [122]	↓Inflammation	

Reducing obesity with dietary restriction and gastric banding [123]	↓Pro-inflammatory activation markers	
Massage therapy in AIDs patients [124]	↑NK cells, CD4, CD8 cells, CD4:CD8 T-cell ratio	
Massage therapy for breast cancer patients [124]	↑NK-cell numbers, lymphocytes	→NK-cell activity
Having adequate sleep [125]	↑Antibody response to vaccination, ↓colds	
Reducing light at night [53]	↑Delayed-type hypersensitivity, bactericidal capacity	
Reducing circadian disruption [55]	↑NK-cell cytotoxicity	
Reduce fatigue due to shift work [126]	↑NK-cell activity, CD16+CD56+ lymphocytes	
Psychological counselling [127]	↑NK-cell cytotoxicity	
Pleasurable experiences: men [128], women [129]	men: ↑NK cells women: ↑Dendritic cells	men: →T cell, B cell, IL-6, Inflammation marker TNF-α
Exclusive breastfeeding (effect on mother) [130]	↑Leukocytes in milk	
Influenza vaccination [131]	↑NK-cell cytotoxicity	
Yellow fever vaccination [132]	↑Cytotoxic T-cells	

Cholera vaccination [133]	↑Antibody response	
Exposure to low-level radiation [84]	↑NK-cell activation	
Short-term exposure to radiofrequency radiation [134]	↑Activation of macrophages	
Radon spa therapy [135]	↑T cells and monocytes	→NK cells, dendritic cells, neutrophils, eosinophils
Ultraviolet blood irradiation [136]	↑Phagocytic activity of human monocytes and granulocytes, activation of neutrophils	
Ozone therapy [137]	↑IFN-γ, IL-2	
Hyperthermia (elevation of body temperature) [138]	↑NK-cell cytotoxic activity	
Whole body vibration exercise [139]	↑Anti-inflammatory (IL-10), ↓pro-inflammatory CRP, TNF-α	
Hyperbaric Oxygen therapy [140]	↓Pro inflammatory cytokines IL-1, IL-6, TNF-α	
Mixed bacteria vaccine [141]	↑IL-6	
Infection [76]	↑NK-cell cytotoxic activity, neutrophil activity, activation of macrophages	
Avoid excessive alcohol consumption during pregnancy [142]	↓Infections in infants	
Breastfeeding (effect on infants) [143]	↑Immunoglobulins, leukocytes	

Massage therapy in preterm infants [144]	↑NK-cell cytotoxicity	→NK-cell numbers
Massage therapy in children with leukemia [124]	↑White blood counts, neutrophil counts	
Contact with livestock, dogs, and cats in the first year of life [145]	↓Respiratory tract infections	
Early vaccination (within 3 months of age) [146]	↓Infection-associated symptoms	

In summary, there are indeed many interventions that can boost the immune system. Two points to note in the Table above are that different interventions enhance different aspects of the immune system and that some interventions do not enhance some components of the immune system.

How can we use all the above information to prevent, treat, and screen for cancers? That will be the subject of the next chapter.

4. CANCER PREVENTION, TREATMENT, AND SCREENING

In the last two chapters, we have seen a considerable amount of evidence to indicate that weakening or suppression of the immune system may be the primary reason for the development of cancer and that different interventions may improve different aspects of the immune system. Now let's discuss how we can use this information to prevent cancer, since it is much better to prevent cancer from occurring than look for a cure after the cancer has been diagnosed.

Prevention of Cancer

Let us examine the effect of physical activity on the cancer mortality rate in adults. Cancer mortality rate has been observed to decrease by about half in the group of adults who had the most physical activity when compared to the group that had the least physical activity (Figure 8) [75].

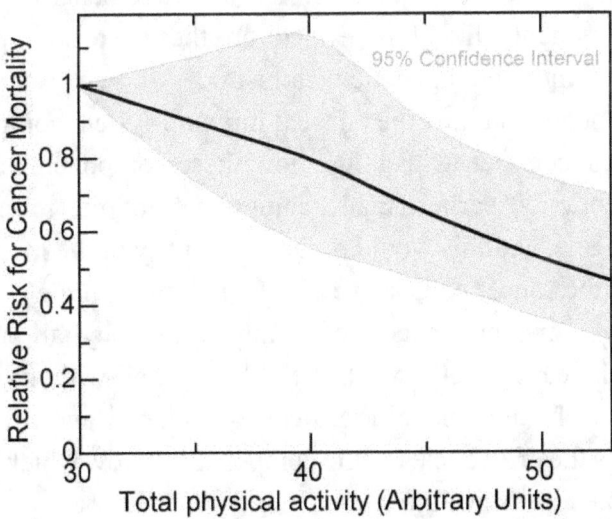

Figure 8. Relative risk of cancer mortality as a function of physical activity. Solid curve represents the estimate of relative risk and the grey shaded area denotes 95% confidence bands. Data from [75].

Why did the cancer mortality rate go down so much with the most physical activity? The explanation, based on what we have seen so far, is that the immune system was enhanced with the increased physical activity and so based on the immune suppression model of cancer, cancer mortality rate went down. However, some of the individuals with the most physical activity did die due to cancer, since their relative risk for cancer mortality rate was not zero but 0.5 (95% CI: 0.3–0.7). Didn't the immune system improve with the high physical activity for these individuals? Why did it not eliminate the cancers? Let's discuss a possible explanation for this now.

Critical Immune System Components

If we examine the various studies that have documented the effect of physical activity or exercise on the immune system, it is clear that different components of the immune system are stimulated in the different studies (see Table 3). Whereas some studies showed improvement in some components of the immune system, others did not show improvement in those components. The improvements in the immune system components likely depended on the exercise type, exercise intensity, age, individual genetic factors, etc.

To understand how the boosted immune system components may reduce the cancers, let us examine how these components change with age. As mentioned earlier, many components of the immune system decline with age, and this would reduce the ability of the immune system to eliminate the cancer cells as we age. In particular, if the efficiencies of some of the components decrease too much, i.e., they fall below certain critical levels, cancer cells would be able to grow without control. We will refer to such components as critical components, and we will refer as critical levels the efficiencies of the components below which cancer cells would be able to grow without control.

Figure 9 shows this concept schematically by plotting the efficiencies of four immune system components labeled A to D as a function of age.

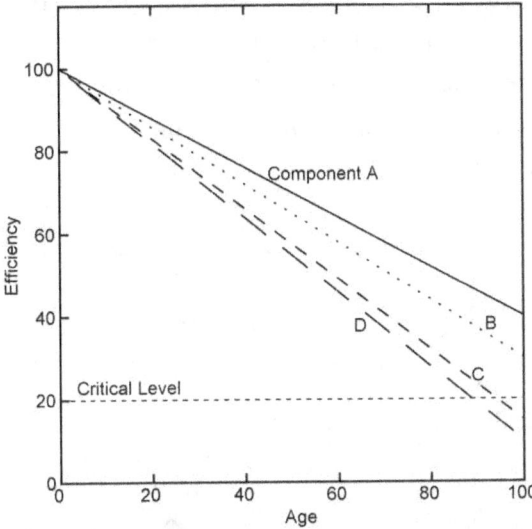

Figure 9. Schematic depiction of the occurrence of fatal cancer due to the linear decline of the efficiencies of the immune system components A, B, C, and D as a function of age. The efficiencies of the components A and B do not fall below the critical level but the efficiencies of the components C and D do fall below the critical level prior to the age of 100. For this example, fatal cancer would occur since two of the efficiencies fall below the critical level.

We will assume that the efficiencies of these components decline linearly with age. Note that I have adjusted the efficiency scale so that the critical level is the same for all the components. Let us assume (to simplify the discussion) that if the efficiencies of two of the components decline below the critical level, the person would develop fatal cancer. We note that the efficiencies of the components A and B do not decline below the critical levels for ages less than 100, and we will assume that the person would die of other causes at the age of 100. Components C and D do decline below the critical level before the age of 100 and so the person would develop fatal cancer.

How Boosting the Immune System Prevents Cancer

How would the cancer risk in this person be affected if he or she utilized some of the immune boosting interventions, e.g. exercise? If exercise improved the performance of the components C and D for the individual so that they did not fall below the critical level, fatal cancer would not occur (Figure 10).

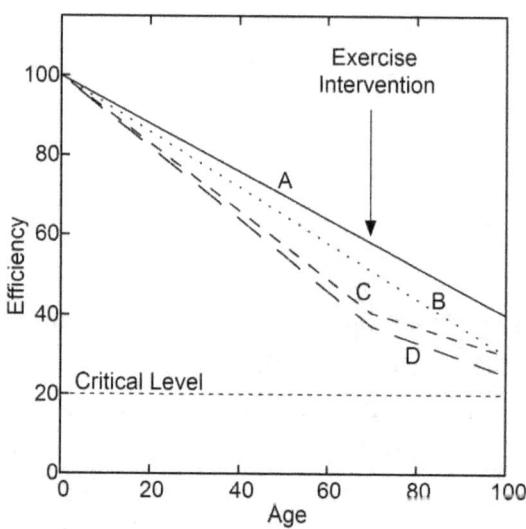

Figure 10. Schematic depiction of exercise intervention preventing fatal cancer. Exercise intervention reduces the rate of decline of the efficiencies of the immune system components C and D, and they do not fall below the critical level. For this example, fatal cancer would not occur since two of the efficiencies do not fall below the critical level.

On the other hand, if the particular types of exercise performed did not improve the critical components C and D but improved the components A and B, cancer fatality would occur in spite of the exercise, since the efficiencies of the components C and D do fall below the critical level (Figure 11).

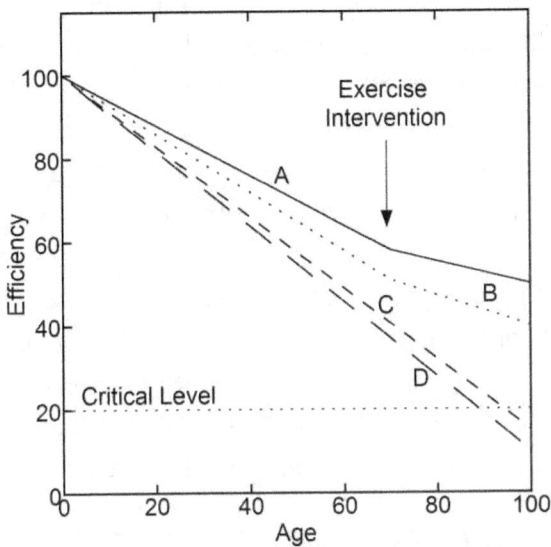

Figure 11. Schematic depiction of exercise intervention not preventing fatal cancer. Exercise intervention reduces the rate of decline of the efficiencies of the immune system components A and B, but does not affect the efficiencies of the components C and D. The efficiencies of the components A and B do not fall below the critical level but the efficiencies of the components C and D do fall below the critical level prior to the age of 100. For this example, fatal cancer would occur since the efficiencies of two of the components decline below the critical level.

This is my hypothesis, based on the immune suppression model of cancer, on why some individuals who exercised at the highest levels succumbed to cancer. This hypothesis needs to be confirmed in further studies. How can these individuals avoid the fatalities due to cancer? If the individuals had utilized other interventions that would improve the performance of the critical components C and D, they could have prevented the deaths from such cancers.

Individualized Interventions to Improve the Immune Response
Actually, we do not know what the critical components of the immune system are for any particular individual, and we also do not know the types of interventions that would enhance the critical components.

However, we do know that different interventions boost different components of the immune system, as noted in the last chapter. Therefore, if we do not want to leave any stone unturned in our effort to prevent cancer, it would make sense to utilize as many of the immune system boosting interventions as practicable. Table 4 provides a list of interventions that would improve the immune response.

Table 4. List of interventions that improve the immune response. Names of organizations or health-related websites that recommend the use of the individual interventions for improving health are shown in parentheses. Frequencies of the interventions mentioned for some of the interventions are suggestions and they may be modified as per user preference.

Exercise – 2.5 hours/week (aerobic and resistance) (American Heart Association)
Be physically active. Limit sitting time (European Code Against Cancer)
Tai chi – 3 times per week for ½ hour (Mayo Clinic)
Dancing – 1/2 hour, 3 times a week (Healthline)
Yoga – 2 sessions per week (WebMD)
Meditation – 3 times per week for 15 minutes (Mayo Clinic)
Rhythmic breathing – 5 times per week for 10 min (Healthline)
Sauna – 3 times per week for 10 min (Healthline)
Taking cold showers – 3 times per week (Healthline)
Forest bathing trips (leisurely trips to the wilderness) 3 times per week for 1 hr. (WebMD)
Vacation at a higher elevation (Berkeley Wellness)
Sunlight exposure (e.g. 15 minutes per day) (National Health Service, UK)
Intermittent Fasting (Healthline)
Calorie restriction – 25% less than the normal amount of food or calories (WebMD)
Fruits and vegetables in diet – 5 to 10 servings per day (European Code Against Cancer)
Turmeric – 1/3 teaspoon per day (Healthline)
Whole grains in diet – 3 servings per day (European Code Against Cancer)
Yogurt – daily (Healthline)

Probiotic foods – daily (Mayo Clinic)
Consumption of deuterium-depleted water (Positive Health Online)
Daily aspirin – 80 mg per day (U.S. Preventive Services Task Force)
Vitamin D supplementation (Healthline)
Statins (Mayo Clinic)
Avoiding high blood sugar levels, for diabetics (CDC)
Reduce red meat in diet to 3 portions or less per week (European Code Against Cancer)
Reducing excessive alcohol use (European Code Against Cancer)
Smoking cessation (European Code Against Cancer)
Reducing obesity with diet, exercise, etc. (European Code Against Cancer)
Gastric banding surgery for weight loss (WebMD)
Bariatric surgery (Cleveland Clinic)
Having adequate sleep (7 hours of sleep per day) (CDC)
Reducing light at night (Harvard Medical)
Ozone therapy (Healthline)
Acupuncture – once per month (Mayo Clinic)
Hyperthermia (NCI)
Hyperbaric oxygen therapy (Johns Hopkins Medicine)
Whole-body vibration exercise (Mayo Clinic)
Short-term exposure to radiofrequency radiation (American Board of Cosmetic Surgery)
Ultraviolet blood irradiation (Science-based Medicine)
Laughter therapy 2 times per week for 1/2 hour (HelpGuide)
Reducing chronic stress with psychological counselling (National Health Service, UK)
Massage – once per month (Mayo Clinic)
Pleasurable experiences (Healthline)
Breastfeeding (for mothers) (European Code Against Cancer)
Annual flu vaccinations (CDC)
Periodic vaccinations as recommended (Tetanus, diphtheria, pertussis, Varicella, Human papillomavirus, Zoster, Measles, mumps, rubella, Pneumococcal, Meningococcal, Hepatitis A, and Hepatitis B) (American Academy of Family Physicians), Travel vaccinations, as recommended (Anthrax, Japanese Encephalitis, Polio, Rabies, Typhoid, Yellow Fever, and

malaria) (CDC, Travel Vaccinations), cholera (CDC), BCG (Tuberculosis) vaccine (CDC)
Mixed bacteria vaccine (Saisei Mirai Clinics)
Exposure to low-level radiation: radon mine (Free-enterprise Radon Health Mine), radon spa (Sanatorium Radon, Khmelnik, Ukraine), radioactive stones (Night Hawk Minerals), radiant beads (Microsec Research & Development), hormesis room (New Energy Research Institute, Japan), radon therapy (Spa Dreams, Europe)
For infants:
Avoidance of excessive alcohol consumption by mothers during pregnancy (CDC)
Breastfeeding for six months or more (American Academy of Pediatrics)
Massage (Mayo Clinic)
Contact with livestock or pets in the first year of life (WebMD)
Childcare attendance (Working Mother)
Childhood vaccinations (CDC)

However, all of the interventions would not be applicable or acceptable for every person. For example, if someone is not a smoker, we cannot ask the person to stop smoking to boost the immune system. If someone is already exercising regularly, we cannot recommend that the person engage in regular exercise to boost the immune system. Also, the interventions may not be acceptable for some people. For example, a smoker may not want to stop smoking. If we recommend to someone that he or she eat more fruits and vegetables to boost the immune system, he or she may not want to do so. Therefore, the list of interventions would need to be individualized based on the individual circumstances and preferences.

One procedure for individualizing the interventions is to ask the individuals questions regarding their lifestyle, circumstances, etc. If any of the above interventions become applicable based on the answers, the individuals would be asked to accept or reject the interventions. The accepted ones would be the individualized interventions for that particular person. I am calling this approach to cancer prevention

"Individualized Interventions to Improve the Immune Response (I^4R)" (Pronunciation key: eye-four-ahr).

Once the individualized interventions are chosen for the individual, a schedule for the use of the interventions should be established by adding some interventions to the schedule each day so that the complete set of individualized interventions would be utilized over the long-term.

How much improvement is needed in the immune system components for preventing cancer? How do we identify the ones most likely to benefit from the I^4R approach for cancer prevention? To answer such questions, let us examine the scope of the cancer problem in the USA.

Preventing Cancer in the Most Vulnerable Group

We saw earlier in Figure 4 that the annual cancer mortality rate in the USA increases with age and is higher for males compared to females. For males, the maximum annual cancer mortality rate is about 2,300 per 100,000 for those over 85 years of age. This implies that around 2.3% of the males over the age of 85 would succumb to cancer during the year, and so 97.7% would not. We have seen earlier that the immune system declines with age, and the highest age group of 85+ would have the lowest immune response but 97.7% of them did not die due to cancer. Why did 2.3% of them succumb to cancer?

Based on the discussions earlier, I would argue that the efficiency of some elements of their immune system had declined to below the critical levels and so the cancer was able to overcome the immune system and grow out of control. But during the previous year, these individuals did not succumb to cancer and so their immune system must have been stronger. The decline in the immune system components in one year is generally a very small amount, and so the efficiencies of their critical immune system components in the previous year would have been low and very close to but above the critical level. If we had somehow identified these individuals (the 2.3% that would succumb to cancer during this year) and had enabled them to boost their immune systems with some interventions during the previous year, cancer could possibly have been prevented in them. **We did not need to boost their immune system by a huge amount, but a small improvement could presumably suffice, provided it is to the critical components of the immune system.** How do we identify the 2.3% who would succumb to cancer? One possibility is to measure the immune system response in all the males over the age of 85, identify the 2.3% of them with the weakest response, and guide them to improve their immune system. Blood tests are available commercially to measure several different aspects of the immune system, and some of these tests may be utilized to measure the immune system response.

Since the immune system has so many components and the immune system responses we measure may not be for the critical components, when using the above procedure, we may miss some individuals that would succumb to cancer. Therefore, it may be better to consider a larger percentage of males over 85, e.g. 10 or 20% of them with the lowest immune response according to our measurements. This is with the expectation that it would include the 2.3% who would succumb to cancer. Once we identify these individuals, we can encourage them to utilize several of the different interventions listed in Table 4 to boost the immune system. If the interventions result in improving the performance of the critical components sufficiently, we may be able to prevent the cancer from occurring in the 2.3% of the males above the age of 85. Is this going to be successful? We need to test this concept in clinical trials to determine if the interventions are effective in reducing the cancer mortality rate in the males above the age of 85.

You may note that the 85+ male population is the group with the highest annual cancer rate, would be the group with the toughest cancer problem to solve, and we have found a procedure that may work for them.

In fact, this method, of identifying the ones with the weakest immune response, can be utilized for the rest of the age groups, and the most vulnerable ones can be prescribed the immune boosting interventions.

Side Effects of the I⁴R Approach

If you examine the different interventions listed in Table 4, you would notice that almost all of them do not have any negative side effects. We should keep in mind that one can indeed be harmed by some of these interventions. For example, whereas yoga is known to be beneficial for health, if it is done incorrectly it can cause injury. Massage with excessive pressure can also cause injury. Aspirin use is associated with reduced cancers, but it can also increase the risk of gastrointestinal bleeding. Therefore, the potential risks of the interventions should be considered prior to the decision on using the individual interventions.

Another aspect of many of these interventions is that they can be beneficial for other aspects of health, in addition to boosting the immune system. For example, vigorous exercise would improve cardiovascular health, and yoga would improve joint health. Therefore, it would make sense to encourage all the population, even those who are not on the lower end of the immune system response, to utilize some of the interventions. Why am I suggesting this?

Why Should Everyone Use the I⁴R?

We know that the immune system response declines with age and some of the lifestyle factors may also decrease the immune response. Therefore, even for those who are not at the low end of the immune response distribution at one time, in later years the immune system may weaken and they may become vulnerable to cancer. If they utilize some immune system boosting interventions, their immune system may be maintained at a high enough level that cancers may not occur.

Another reason to start the interventions in those who have a strong immune system is that some of the interventions may reduce the aging-related decline in the immune system [95].

Cancer Screening

The method described above, of measuring the immune system response to identify the ones with the lowest levels of the immune system response, should be studied as a cancer screening technique. Based on the immune suppression model of cancer, such individuals would face an increased risk of cancer. Therefore, screening in this manner and the resulting interventions may prevent the cancers from developing in these individuals.

One caveat for this method of screening is that blood tests may not determine the efficiency of the immune system components that are not circulating in the blood. Therefore, the screening process may not identify all the vulnerable people. It may be best to encourage all the members of the public to undertake some immune boosting interventions and to gradually increase the number of such interventions as they age, in order to protect themselves from cancer.

How many of the interventions should one use? With the knowledge gained from following up of the participants of the I^4R clinical trials, we would be able to establish guidelines on how many interventions would be ideal. If one has a higher risk of cancer based on genetic and lifestyle factors, it may be advisable to use more interventions. Counseling should be provided to all the individuals based on their estimated cancer risk regarding the recommended set of immune boosting interventions.

I^4R approach for the Treatment of Early-Stage Cancer

Now let's discuss how we can treat patients who are diagnosed with early-stage cancer, either due to observed symptoms, incidental findings from imaging, or from using the traditional cancer screening programs. Detection of early-stage cancer through cancer screening programs (or as incidental findings from imaging studies) does not necessarily imply that a normal cell has just transformed into a cancer cell and has started multiplying, since almost everyone has cancer cells or precancerous cells in their bodies [25]. Detection of early-stage cancer through screening may more likely imply that we have identified a dormant cancer. Such a covert cancer may not develop into a real cancer and it may resolve itself [147]. Detection of early-stage cancer through symptoms (e.g. a lump observed at a location where there were no lumps weeks or months earlier) may not imply a normal cell has just transformed into a cancer cell and has developed into a detectable lump. Based on the immune suppression model of cancer, it may more likely imply that the immune system function has declined during the recent period allowing the already existing cancer cells to multiply and develop into a lump. Why did the immune system decline? It likely declined due to factors such as lifestyle and aging. Therefore, if the immune system is enhanced, it may be able to control the cancer cells and eliminate them or send them back into a covert state.

In view of this situation, early-stage cancers should be treated by enhancing the immune system with the I⁴R approach. The immune system response should be measured before and after the interventions to verify the enhancement of the immune system. If the observed cancer symptoms begin to regress, the immune boosting interventions should be continued. If the cancer does not regress in spite of the immune enhancing interventions, additional interventions should be prescribed. If there is still no reduction of cancer, traditional methods would need to be used to eliminate the cancer. I am hopeful that for most individuals, the I⁴R approach would eliminate the early-stage cancers and the traditional cancer treatments may not be needed. This needs to be studied through clinical trials.

The Benefits of Traditional Cancer Screening
in the I⁴R Approach to Cancer

When someone is diagnosed with early-stage cancer through the traditional cancer screening programs, and if we respond by using the I⁴R approach, the resulting immune boosting interventions would have the potential to improve the health of the individual, in comparison to someone who did not undergo the screening. In addition, based on the immune suppression model of cancer, the interventions may eliminate the early-stage cancer, and this can be confirmed in the follow-up examinations some time following the immune boosting interventions. In this manner, the traditional cancer screenings for a few types of cancers can play an important role by providing a warning to patients about the possible weakness of their immune system and by providing them the motivation to undertake the immune boosting interventions, improving their health, and possibly eliminating the early-stage cancers. This concept needs to be studied in clinical trials.

I^4R Approach for the Treatment of Late-Stage Cancer

How should we deal with the late-stage cancers? Would immune boosting interventions be sufficient to cure the late-stage cancers? Over a hundred years ago, Dr. William Coley made the observation that in several cancer patients who had large-size tumors and metastatic disease, the tumors disappeared following the occurrence of erysipelas, a bacterial skin infection [148]. Based on this observation, he decided to try treating patients with a mixed bacteria vaccine, popularly known as Coley's toxins. Some of the cancer patients he treated had complete remission of cancer [149]. A possible explanation for the complete cure of these cancers is that the infections boosted the immune system, and the boosted immune system eliminated the cancers. The successful examples of Coley's treatments indicate that late stage cancers may also be successfully treated by boosting the immune system. Therefore, the I^4R approach should be tested in clinical trials with late-stage cancers also. As many of the applicable interventions should be used as feasible, in order to improve the chance that the boosted immune system would eliminate the cancer cells. Clinical trials are needed to determine what fraction of the late-stage cancer patients would benefit from the I^4R approach.

Use of the I^4R Approach between Cancer Diagnosis and the Beginning of Treatment

The I^4R approach may also be utilized by patients who are diagnosed with cancer and are waiting for the traditional treatments to begin. When someone is diagnosed with cancer, and the standard treatments are being planned, it may take several weeks or even a few months to complete the additional diagnostic tests and prepare for the treatments. It would also be a good idea to obtain a second opinion on the cancer diagnosis, since sometimes the diagnosis is in error [150]. For deciding on the traditional cancer treatment plan also, it may be useful to obtain a second opinion as it may result in a change in the treatment plan [151].

While waiting for these additional investigations and second opinions to be completed, it may be advisable (based on the immune suppression model of cancer) for the patient to select the interventions that are applicable and acceptable to him/her from those listed in Table 4, and start the chosen interventions as soon as possible, under the supervision of a qualified health-care professional, as part of a clinical trial or based on the recommendations of health-related websites, e.g., those listed in Table 4. Sometime after the interventions, and before the treatments are scheduled to begin, another evaluation of the patient's cancer status should be done, using the method most appropriate for the type and stage of cancer. It is possible that the boosted immune system would control the cancers and the observed symptoms (cancer biomarkers, extent of metastasis, size of lump, PSA level, etc.) may decrease by the time of the scheduled treatment. If this is observed, it may be possible to defer the standard treatments, continue the immune boosting interventions, and monitor the cancer status closely. If the symptoms continue to recede and disappear, it would indicate that the I^4R approach has worked. If the cancer symptoms re-appear, additional immune boosting interventions may be prescribed.

This approach, of using the I^4R approach between the cancer diagnosis and the beginning of treatment should be studied in clinical trials to determine if sufficient reduction of cancer symptoms can be achieved with the interventions and whether the continuation of the I^4R approach would prevent the cancer from re-appearing in the patient.

You may wonder, if a few weeks or months of the I^4R approach interventions are going to be sufficient to show a reduction of the cancer symptoms in order to determine if the interventions have been effective. PET/CT scan performed two weeks after the beginning of targeted therapy (a type of cancer treatment) has been shown to provide a reliable indication that the targeted therapy is working, obviating the need for chemotherapy in breast cancer patients [152]. Early PSA response, four weeks after the initiation of treatment with androgen pathway inhibitors, has been shown to be a good indication that the treatment of prostate cancer is working [153]. Based on such observations, evaluation of the patient a few weeks or months after starting the I^{4}R approach interventions may provide a valuable indication on whether the interventions are working. This needs to be studied in clinical trials.

The I^{4}R Approach Following the Traditional Cancer Treatments

A problem faced by many cancer patients following the traditional cancer treatments is cancer recurrence. Another problem faced by such patients is the increased risk of second cancers. Based on the immune suppression model of cancer, the occurrence of both of these problems may be reduced by the use of the I^{4}R approach after the completion of the traditional cancer treatments. This should be studied in clinical trials.

The I^{4}R Approach Should Not be a Brief Intervention but a Change Adopted for Lifetime

Let us assume that someone uses the I^{4}R approach for cancer and it results in eliminating the cancer symptoms. This should not result in the discontinuance of the immune boosting interventions because the immune system would likely become weaker making the person susceptible to cancer again. On the other hand, when the success of the I^{4}R approach is noted, the interventions should be continued, and it would be advisable to gradually increase the number of immune boosting interventions as the person ages, to counteract the anticipated aging-related decline in the immune system. Counseling should be provided to cancer patients about the optimum set of immune boosting interventions based on an assessment of their age, family history, lifestyle, genetics, and other risk factors.

Cancer Prevention in Genetically Susceptible Individuals

Individuals with certain mutations are known to have an elevated risk of cancer. For example, females with the BRCA mutations have an increased risk of breast and ovarian cancers. Many of them currently undergo surgeries for the removal of the breasts, ovaries, and fallopian tubes to reduce the risk of the cancers [154], and such surgeries are known to reduce the mortality rate in the BRCA mutation carriers [155]. Would it be possible to reduce the cancer risk in such individuals under the I^4R approach without the surgeries? Would the immune boosting interventions reduce their cancer risk?

Increased physical activity, which boosts the immune system, has been observed to reduce the risk of breast cancer in BRCA mutation carriers [156]. Another study has shown that reduction of body weight, which would boost the immune system, resulted in reducing breast cancer risk in BRCA mutation carriers [157]. Thus, these immune boosting interventions did reduce the breast cancer risk in such patients. Other immune boosting interventions may also reduce their cancer risk. Would additional immune boosting interventions be sufficient to eliminate the risk of breast and ovarian cancers in the BRCA mutation carriers? Clinical trials are needed to answer this question. If the answer turns out to be in the affirmative, the surgeries that are currently performed to reduce the risk of cancers in the BRCA mutation carriers may possibly be avoided.

Immune System Evading Cancers

How can we deal with the immune system evading cancers under the I^4R approach? Since the I^4R approach boosts the immune system through multiple methods, many components of the immune system would be boosted, and so the immune system may be able to overcome the immune resistance and eliminate the immune system evading cancers. Based on this concept, my hypothesis is that the I^4R approach would be effective in eliminating the immune system evading cancers. If the clinical trials of the I^4R approach show that it is effective in preventing and treating all cancers, this hypothesis would be confirmed. If the clinical trials show that a certain fraction of the cancers are not prevented or treated effectively with the I^4R approach, traditional cancer treatments would need to be utilized for such cancers.

If the I⁴R approach is followed for cancer prevention, the problem of the immune system evading cancers would be reduced, because the boosted immune system would eliminate more of the cancer cells and reduce the number of cancer cells that are in an equilibrium state when the immune system evading cancer cells tend to develop [35], as explained in Chapter 2. In addition, some of the recommended interventions, e.g. exercise [158] and low-dose radiation [159], would boost the cellular defenses such as antioxidants and DNA repair enzymes. These defenses would reduce the DNA damage and mutations in the body, reducing the chance that cancer cells are formed. Studies have shown that following regular exercise, reduced DNA damage has been observed in humans [158]. **Studies have also shown that following exposure to low-level radiation, the mutation rates are reduced in fruit flies [160] and in mice [161-162].** In a study of the population living in Ramsar, Iran, when the lymphocytes of the population were exposed to very high radiation levels, reduced chromosomal damage was observed in the lymphocytes of the population living in the areas with elevated background radiation levels in comparison to those living in the areas with normal background radiation levels [163]. This indicates that the lymphocytes of the population in the areas with elevated background radiation levels may have higher defenses. **In view of these types of data, interventions such as exercise and low-level radiation may reduce the amount of DNA damage and mutations, reducing the chance for the formation of the immune system evading cancers.** This needs to be studied in clinical trials.

Use of the I⁴R Approach in the Absence of Clinical Trials

Several of the immune-boosting interventions listed in Table 4 are recommended by professional organizations such as American Institute for Cancer Research (AICR) and Centers for Disease Control and Prevention (CDC) for reducing cancer risk. Other listed interventions are known to improve health in other ways, and are recommended by professional organizations or health-related websites, as listed in the Table. Even without participating in clinical trials, individuals may utilize these interventions based on such recommendations, after consulting with their qualified health-care professionals.

In summary, it may be possible to prevent and treat cancer by boosting the immune system using the I^4R approach, i.e. by using the individualized interventions to improve the immune response. Clinical trials are needed to determine if the I^4R approach is effective in preventing and treating cancers.

The I^4R approach that I have described in this chapter is quite different from the traditional approach for dealing with cancer. You may wonder if there are any advantages in using the I^4R approach. That will be the subject of the next chapter.

5. ADVANTAGES OF THE I4R APPROACH

We saw in the last chapter that "Individualized Interventions to Improve the Immune Response", the I^4R approach, may be useful for preventing and treating cancer. How does the I^4R approach compare to the current approach in dealing with cancer? Table 5 lists the differences between the current approach and the I^4R approach for different aspects of the cancer field.

Table 5. Comparison of the current approach to cancer with the proposed I^4R approach.

Aspect	Current Approach	The I^4R Approach
Cancer Screening	Available and recommended (by the CDC, for example) for a few of the cancers. Other cancers, which are unscreened, can grow undetected.	Immune system measurements are conducted to identify those with the weakest immune response. Designed to determine the susceptibility for all the cancers.
Consequence of detection of early-stage cancer	Cancer treatments with potential for adverse side effects.	Beneficial immune boosting interventions.
Consequence of overdiagnosis (Diagnosis of early-stage cancer which would not develop into a real cancer)	Overdiagnosis would result in treatments that have a potential for adverse side effects, and so overdiagnosis may be harmful to patients.	Overdiagnosis would result in immune boosting interventions that have very few adverse side effects but many beneficial effects. Therefore, overdiagnosis would be beneficial to patients.

Slow-growing cancers	Patients are not pleased with watchful waiting [164].	Patients can be proactive and take actions based on the I^4R approach.
Adverse side effects of treatments	Minor and major adverse side effects. Deterioration of quality of life.	Few adverse side effects are expected. Many of the interventions used in the I^4R approach would improve health.
Cancer risk from treatments	Increased risk of second cancers from radiation therapy [165] and chemotherapy [166]	Decreased risk of second cancers expected from the I^4R approach.

As seen in the above Table, the I^4R approach overcomes several of the disadvantages of the present approach to cancer, and is much more patient-friendly.

In summary, the comparison of the I^4R approach with the current approach to cancer indicates that the I^4R approach holds many advantages for cancer patients. You may ask how well the I^4R approach would be in preventing and treating cancer. That will be the subject of the next chapter.

6. ESTIMATING THE EFFECTIVENESS OF THE I4R APPROACH

Though the I^{4}R approach has not been studied in clinical trials, there is a considerable amount of data on the beneficial health effects of individual immune boosting interventions, both for reducing the mortality in cancer patients and for reducing the cancer incidence and mortality for the general public.

Past Studies of Individual Immune Boosting Interventions for Cancer Patients

Many of the immune boosting interventions have resulted in reduction of mortality in cancer patients, as indicated in Table 6. The Table lists the percentage reduction in the mortality rate observed in the cancer patients following the interventions, and the 95% confidence intervals (CIs). The 95% CIs give a range of values that one can be 95% certain that it includes the true mean value.

Table 6. Reduction of mortality rates observed in the cancer patients following the individual immune system boosting interventions.

Immune system boosting intervention	Percentage reduction in the mortality rate of the cancer patients with 95% CIs shown in parentheses
Increased physical activity in men diagnosed with any cancer (highest activity vs. lowest activity) [167]	48% (35–58%)
Plant-based diet in colorectal cancer patients [168]	38% (17–53%)
Smoking cessation [169]	15% (3–24%)
Daily aspirin [170]	19% (11–27%)
Psychological support that led to decline in depression symptoms in breast cancer patients [171]	40% (14–59%)

Cholera vaccination in prostate cancer patients [172]	47% (31–59%)
Hyperthermia for cervical cancer patients [173]	40% (5–62%)
Repeated exposure to low-level radiation for non-Hodgkin's lymphoma patients [174]	44% (8–80%)¶

¶Note: The percentage reduction shown is with reference to the patients who underwent chemotherapy. Hence, the percentage reduction in the mortality rate attributable to low-level radiation exposures would be much larger.

Past Studies of the Effect of Immune Boosting Interventions on Cancer in the Public

Many of the immune boosting interventions have been observed to result in reduced cancer incidence (Table 7) and reduced cancer mortality (Table 8) in the general population.

Table 7: Immune system boosting interventions and their effects on the cancer incidence rates in the public. The first column lists the interventions and the second column indicates the percentage reduction in the cancer incidence rates for all cancers that has been observed in the population group having the interventions.

Immune system boosting intervention	Percentage reduction in the cancer incidence rate. 95% CIs are shown in parentheses
Physical activity, 60-90 minutes per day [75]	16% (2–28%)
Men, smoking cessation for 21+ years [175]	36% (29–43%)
Women, smoking cessation for 11+ years [175]	30% (4–49%)

Statin (Atorvastatin) use in patients with Type 2 diabetes [176]	71% (12–91%)
Reduction of 3 servings of red meat per week [177]	8% (6–11%)
Reducing obesity with bariatric surgery [83]	33% (26–40%)
Exposure to low-level radiation [178]	16% (5–26%)
Contact with livestock in the first year of life [179]	35% (15–50%)[§]
Contact with dogs in the first year of life [179]	8% (1–14%)[§]
Contact with cats in the first year of life [179]	13% (6–20%)[§]
Any vaccination in the first year [180]	42% (9–64%)[¶]

[¶] Childhood leukemias

[§] Childhood acute lymphoblastic leukemias

Table 8. Immune system boosting interventions and their effects on the cancer mortality rates in the public. The first column lists the interventions and the second column indicates the percentage reduction in the cancer mortality rates for all cancers that has been observed in the population group having the interventions.

Immune system boosting intervention	Percentage reduction in the cancer mortality rate. 95% CIs are shown in parentheses
Physical activity (highest activity vs. lowest) [75]	55% (32–72%)
Smoking cessation [181]	38% (36-40%)
Fruits and vegetables 500 gm per day vs. none [182]	13% (10–16%)
Statin Use [183]	15% (9–17%)

Reduction of 3 servings of red meat per week [177]	8% (6–11%)
Annual flu vaccinations [81]	26% (14–36%)
Vitamin D supplementation [184]	13% (4–21%)
Exposure to low-level radiation [185]	15% (8–22%)

The data in the above Tables 7 and 8 indicate that substantial reduction in the cancer incidence and mortality rates have been observed following these interventions in the general population, and the data in Table 6 indicate that substantial reduction of mortality rate has been observed in the cancer patients following the interventions. Many of the other interventions listed in Table 4 also may lead to similar reductions.

How can we use the above information to reduce the cancer rates in the general population? Let us consider the level of leisure-time physical activity of adults in the USA. It has been reported that 34% of the adults are physically inactive [186]. Let us imagine that we are able to convince the adults who are inactive to become physically active at a high level. Based on the data in Table 8, there would be a 55% reduction in their cancer mortality rate. This would result in 55% x 34%, i.e. 19% reduction of cancer mortality in the whole population.

This example illustrates the high potential for reducing cancer mortality rate by following the I⁴R approach, considering that the use of just one intervention on a fraction of the population may reduce the cancer mortality rate by 19% in the population. Of course, it is not likely that we would be successful in changing the lifestyle of the inactive adult population. However, there are many other interventions in Table 4 that are not of lifestyle type, and compliance with these interventions could be achievable on a large scale. For example, if the advisory bodies examine and validate the evidence for the cancer preventive and therapeutic effects of low-level radiation, as explained in Appendix A, the use of low-level radiation can be tested in clinical trials for cancer prevention, and if the clinical trials confirm the cancer preventive effect of low-level radiation, its widespread utilization may reduce the cancer mortality rate by about 20 percent, based on the data from the available studies [85].

To illustrate the impact of utilizing multiple immune boosting interventions, let us consider a hypothetical country in which we assume that each of the interventions listed in Table 8 is applicable to the population and all of the population agrees to utilize the interventions. Under these assumptions, the cancer mortality rate reduction factor, the factor by which mortality rate would reduce with the use of the intervention, can be calculated for each of the interventions. As an example, for physical activity, considering that the percentage reduction in the cancer mortality rate with increased physical activity was 55% (Table 8), the cancer mortality rate reduction factor would be (100-55.5)/100, i.e. 0.45. Calculating the mortality rate reduction factor for the other interventions in a similar manner, and multiplying all the mortality rate reduction factors for the interventions listed in Table 8, we can estimate that the cancer mortality rate in the public may be reduced by a factor of 0.10, i.e. by 90% with the use of all the eight interventions by the population. If more of the interventions listed in Table 4 are utilized, a larger reduction of cancer mortality rate may be achievable.

A similar calculation using the data in Table 6 would show that for cancer patients, the use of the 8 listed interventions may reduce the mortality rate of the cancer patients by 98%. Additional interventions from Table 4 may further reduce the mortality rate in the cancer patients. Whereas these are hypothetical calculations for an imaginary country, they do illustrate the cancer reducing potential of using multiple immune boosting interventions for those who choose to use them.

Thus, there is a high potential for reducing the adverse impact of cancer in the public and in the cancer patients with the use of the I^4R approach. This needs to be studied in clinical trials.

Synergistic Effect of Multiple Immune-Boosting Interventions in Preventing and Treating Cancer

It is possible that some of the individual immune boosting interventions are not sufficient by themselves to elevate the efficiencies of the critical components of the immune system above the critical levels. For such cases, the combined effect of multiple interventions may be sufficient to elevate them above the critical levels. If this occurs, there could be a cancer preventive or therapeutic effect with the multiple interventions even though individually the interventions did not produce such an effect. Clinical trials are needed to determine if there is such a synergistic effect from utilizing the multiple interventions. If the answer is in the affirmative, it would provide additional justification for the use of multiple immune boosting interventions for cancer prevention and treatment.

In summary, based on the existing data for the effect of the individual immune boosting interventions on the outcomes of the cancer patients and the general public, the I^4R approach holds the potential to reduce the mortality rates for the cancer patients and to reduce the cancer incidence and mortality rates for the general public by large amounts.

In view of its advantages as discussed in the last Chapter and the potential beneficial effects discussed in the present chapter, it is clear that the I^4R approach should be studied in clinical trials to determine if the patient outcomes with the approach are as good as or better than the current standard of care. How can we facilitate the clinical trials of the I^4R approach? That will be the subject of the next chapter.

7. CLINICAL TRIALS OF THE I4R APPROACH

The I^{4}R approach that I have described in the last few chapters is quite different from the current well-established approach to cancer that has been followed worldwide for many decades. Clinical trials are needed to validate the I^{4}R approach to cancer.

Facilitating the Clinical Trials of the I^{4}R Approach

Since there are a large variety of immune-boosting interventions, it would be useful to set up new enterprises known as I4R Centers where all or most of the immune boosting interventions are made available. Such I4R Centers would facilitate the clinical trials of the I^{4}R approach by making it convenient for the public and patients to utilize the interventions without requiring travel to different locations for different interventions. Early investors in this type of enterprises may have a considerable advantage due to the experience and reputation gained from the operation of the I4R Centers. If the clinical trials of the I^{4}R approach provide good results and the approach is adopted by the medical community in the future, there would be a tremendous potential for the growth of such enterprises, since the approach would be needed and used not only by the cancer patients for cancer treatment but also by the entire population for cancer prevention.

You may have noted that a large number of the interventions to boost the immune system are lifestyle changes. It is well known from previous studies that it is not easy to achieve lifestyle changes on a consistent basis [187]. Therefore, it is important that we make full use of the non-lifestyle-based interventions. For one of the non-lifestyle-based interventions, low-level radiation, currently there are major hurdles for studying it in clinical trials. Though this is just one of the immune boosting interventions, it has been observed to have cancer preventive [185] and therapeutic [174] effects in past studies. Considering that cancer has been a tough nut to crack, it would make sense to not leave any stone unturned in our efforts to solve the cancer problem. Therefore, it is important that we arm ourselves with everything we can and implement this intervention in clinical trials, and utilize it if it is found to be beneficial. Appendix A discusses the hurdles facing low-level radiation as an intervention and how the study of this intervention may be enabled.

Now let us discuss the types of clinical trials that can be conducted to determine the usefulness of the I⁴R approach.

Cancer Treatment Clinical Trials

In these clinical trials, eligible patients would be randomly assigned to an I⁴R group or a control group. The patients in the I⁴R group would be asked to choose the interventions that are applicable and acceptable to them from the interventions listed in Table 4. Once the individualized interventions are chosen by a patient, a schedule for the use of the interventions would be established by adding some of the interventions to the schedule each day so that the complete set of individualized interventions would be utilized over the long-term.

The patients would be given the selected individualized interventions. Immune system measurements would be conducted using blood samples collected from the patients at the beginning of the study and periodically during the trial period. The patients in the control group would be offered the traditional cancer treatments appropriate for the type and stage of cancer. Patients in both the groups would be followed up using the various diagnostic scans, physical examinations, etc. as appropriate and the status of the disease would be determined for the patients in each group. From such data, the effectiveness of the I⁴R approach for treating cancer patients would be determined.

Pilot Clinical Trials of the I⁴R Approach for Cancer Treatment

My view is that based on the evidence presented in Table 6, head-to-head comparison cancer treatment clinical trials between the I⁴R approach and the traditional approach are justifiable. However, since the I⁴R approach is an untested method, there may be reluctance to use it in such head-to-head comparison clinical trials. In order to address such concerns, the initial pilot clinical trials may be designed for situations such as the following where the traditional treatments are not being given:

a. Patients undergoing watchful waiting for prostate cancer or other cancers. For a group of such patients, the immune boosting interventions based on the I^4R approach can be prescribed and the outcomes of such patients can be compared to a group undergoing the traditional watchful waiting only.

b. Cancer patients for whom there is likely to be a substantial time period between the diagnoses and the beginning of the treatments due to the additional tests that need to be conducted or due to the process of obtaining second opinions on the diagnoses or the treatments. For a group of such patients, immune boosting interventions can be prescribed, and the status of the disease can be evaluated sometime prior to the beginning of the cancer treatments. If no regression of the cancer is observed, the traditional treatments can be started. If regression of the disease is observed following the use of the I^4R approach, the traditional treatments may be deferred, the immune boosting interventions can be continued, and the patient's status can be monitored closely.

c. Patients who refuse the traditional cancer treatments. A small percentage of the cancer patients are known to refuse the recommended standard treatments [188-189]. Studies of such patients have shown that those who refuse the traditional treatments have worse outcomes [190-191]. For a group of such patients, immune boosting interventions based on the I^4R approach can be prescribed, and the outcomes compared to equivalent patients that undergo the standard treatments.

One advantage of these categories of patients is that they would not be undergoing any traditional cancer treatments during the course of the I^4R interventions and so the benefits of the I^4R approach can be assessed without any interference from the traditional treatments.

If the pilot clinical trials show that the I^4R approach results in better patient outcomes than the traditional approach, it would justify detailed clinical trials of head-to-head comparisons between the I^4R approach and the traditional approach.

The I^4R Approach May Transform Temporary Cure of Present Treatments into a Permanent Cure

Many of the traditional cancer treatments are successful in the short-term but fail in the long-term as the tumors develop resistance, i.e. they do not respond to the treatments after some time and the tumors recur [192-198]. The use of the I^4R approach shortly after the completion of the traditional cancer treatments may boost the immune system sufficiently to prevent the re-occurrence of the cancers, and so provide a permanent cure of cancer. This needs to be studied in clinical trials.

Now let us discuss the clinical trials of cancer prevention.

Cancer Prevention Clinical Trials

In these clinical trials, eligible individuals would be randomly assigned to an I^4R group or a control group. The individuals in the I^4R group would be asked to choose the interventions that are applicable and acceptable to them from the interventions listed in Table 4. Once the interventions are chosen by an individual, a schedule for the use of the interventions would be established by adding some of the interventions to the schedule each day so that the complete set of individualized interventions would be utilized over the long-term.

The individuals would be given the selected, individualized interventions according to the schedule. Immune system measurements would be conducted using blood samples collected from the individuals at the beginning of the study and periodically during the trial period. The health status of the subjects would be monitored and recorded periodically. Comparison of the cancer outcomes of the I^4R group with the control group would be used to assess the effectiveness of the I^4R approach in preventing cancer.

Cancer Screening Clinical Trials

Measurements of the immune system response would be performed for all the members of the general public in order to identify and select the individuals who have the lowest immune system response. The selected subjects would be randomly assigned to an I⁴R group or a control group. The subjects in the I⁴R group would be offered the individualized interventions to improve the immune response. The health status of the participants would be monitored and recorded periodically. The subjects in both the groups would be offered the traditional cancer screenings. The cancer rates in both the groups would be compared to determine whether the I⁴R approach is effective in preventing cancers in comparison to the traditional cancer screenings alone.

Standardizations Prior to the Widespread Clinical Trials

If the pilot clinical trials of the I⁴R approach show that the results are as good as or better than the traditional approach, widespread clinical trials of the I⁴R approach would be justified. Prior to the start of such widespread clinical trials, interested professionals from the various institutions should form a standardization committee, and it should establish the standards for the immune boosting interventions and the immune system measurements. Thereafter, any clinical trials of the I⁴R approach should be urged to use these standards for the immune system measurements and the immune boosting interventions. In this manner, the data from the various clinical trials at the different institutions would be consistent and could be combined into a single database for consistent interpretation.

Registries for the Clinical Trials of the I⁴R Approach

National and international registries should be established for the clinical trials of the I⁴R approach so that the data from all the clinical trials can be collected into a single database. The data accumulated in the registries can be useful in evaluating the relative effectiveness of the different combinations of the immune boosting interventions for cancer prevention and treatment.

Examples of Questions That Need to be answered in the Clinical Trials

If the pilot clinical trials give promising results, many more clinical trials would be needed to answer the questions such as the following:

- Can the recurrence of cancer and the occurrence of second cancers be reduced with the I^4R approach in the patients who have been treated for cancer through the traditional methods?
- Can early-stage cancers and late-stage cancers be treated effectively with the I^4R approach?
- Which interventions or combinations of interventions are the most effective for cancer prevention and treatment?
- Is the recurrence of cancer avoided when cancer is treated using the I^4R approach?
- Does the I^4R approach for cancer prevention reduce the occurrence of the immune system evading cancers?
- Is the I^4R approach effective in treating the immune system evading cancers?
- Is the I^4R approach effective in preventing cancers in the individuals who are genetically susceptible to cancer, e.g. BRCA mutation carriers?
- Do vaccinations other than the flu vaccination have a cancer preventive and/or therapeutic effect?
- Are non-lifestyle-based interventions sufficient to prevent and treat cancer?
- What fraction of cancers is prevented by the I^4R approach?
- What fraction of cancers is treated effectively by the I^4R approach?

As you can see, a considerable amount of research needs to be done in the form of clinical trials to validate the I^4R approach, determine its limitations, and to optimize its use. Therefore, it is important that the pilot clinical trials are started promptly so that if the results justify, the detailed clinical trials can be conducted to answer the questions such as those listed above.

I am hopeful that following the detailed clinical trials, the I^{4}R approach would be found to be effective in preventing cancer, and in case cancer occurs, it would be found to be very effective in treating it with few adverse side effects, with the potential to revolutionize the cancer field.

Since the I^{4}R approach is quite different from the currently well-established approach to cancer, there may be hesitation in conducting the clinical trials of the approach. Strong public support would be very helpful in enabling the clinical trials of the I^{4}R approach. You may wonder why you, the reader of the book, should support the clinical trials. That will be the subject of the next chapter.

8. HERE IS MY PITCH

Our Current Approach to Cancer is Not Satisfactory

Cancer is a serious problem in our present society, and the reported advances over the past several decades have not led to a large reduction in the cancer mortality rates (Figure 1). Also, two decades of advances in cancer treatments have led to only a modest reduction in the 5-year mortality rates of metastatic cancer patients (Table 1).

Other Approaches Such as the I⁴R Approach Should be studied in Clinical Trials

Since our current approach to cancer has led to only a modest progress in the war on cancer, it is incumbent upon us to explore other approaches which have the potential to provide better results. The basis for the approach to cancer that I have proposed in this book is the observation that cancer risk increases tremendously when the immune system is suppressed in young individuals [32,34]. Based on this, I have proposed the hypotheses that the main reason for the development of most cancers is the weakening or suppression of the immune system [36], and that cancer develops when the efficiencies of some components of the immune system fall below certain critical levels. Therefore, cancer may be prevented and treated by boosting these critical components so that their efficiencies are maintained above the critical levels. The I⁴R approach, i.e., "Individualized Interventions to Improve the Immune Response", since it uses multiple immune boosting interventions, would boost many components of the immune system, and so is likely to boost the critical components and have a cancer preventive and therapeutic effect. The available evidence on the individual immune boosting interventions indicates that the use of multiple interventions under the I⁴R approach may result in a substantial reduction of the cancer risk for the public and a large reduction of mortality rates for the cancer patients (Tables 6, 7, and 8). Therefore, it is important that we study the I⁴R approach in clinical trials. Success in preventing and treating cancer using the I^4R approach in the clinical trials would validate the above hypotheses and the I^4R approach.

The Current Standard of Care Should Continue to be used for Treating Cancer Patients

Notwithstanding the strong reasons I have given for supporting the I^4R approach to cancer in clinical trials, **unless and until the clinical trials validate the I^4R approach and the medical community has adopted it, the current standard of care should continue to be used for treating the cancer patients since it is the best approach we have at present**, and outcomes have been much worse for patients who have refused the traditional treatments.

How You Can Help to Advance the I^4R Approach to Cancer

If you appreciate the many advantages of the I^4R approach for the cancer patients and the public, I would request that you take one or more of the following actions:

1. Visit the book website: https://bit.ly/2E1JHxj and express your support for the I^4R approach by answering the survey there on the approach. This is a very important step that you can take to support the I^4R approach, since it is an unconventional approach and a strong public support for the concept is crucial for enabling the clinical trials of the approach and its potential adoption by the medical community.
2. Spread the word about the book and the advantages of the I^4R approach by informing your friends and colleagues via email, social media, etc. Increased publicity would generate more interest in the approach and would facilitate the initiation of the clinical trials of the approach in many institutions.
3. Inform your family physician about this book and the I^4R approach so that he or she can guide you as well as other patients in its use for cancer prevention and treatment.

4. Inform opinion leaders that you know regarding the book and the I^{4}R approach so that they can in turn inform others about the approach.

5. Set up an I4R Center in your neighborhood to provide all or most of the I^{4}R interventions in one location.

6. Support clinical trials of the I4R approach. If you are interested in supporting the clinical trials, please contact me via email so that we can discuss how you can help.

The potential revolution in the cancer field described in this book may be achieved if concerted efforts are made by a large number of interested people. I wish to thank you, the readers of the book, for playing your part in helping to enable this potential revolution.

Why Everyone Who is concerned about Cancer should Read this Book

Now let me discuss why anyone who is concerned about a possible cancer diagnosis in the future and the resulting adverse consequences should read this book. If someone is diagnosed with cancer and has already read the book and has become familiar with the I^{4}R approach, he or she would know to utilize the applicable interventions listed in Table 4 under the supervision of a qualified health-care professional, as part of a clinical trial or based on the recommendations of the websites listed in Table 4. If these interventions are started very shortly after the cancer diagnosis, there may be sufficient time for the effects of the interventions to manifest themselves in the form of reduced cancer symptoms, before the scheduled beginning of the traditional treatments. If these are observed, it may be possible to defer the cancer treatments, continue the immune boosting interventions, and monitor closely for the cancer symptoms. Thus, the adverse consequences following the cancer diagnosis may be deferred and possibly avoided because of reading the book, being prepared, and taking prompt actions. An even better consequence of reading the book may be that the readers would be motivated and start utilizing some of the immune boosting interventions under the I^{4}R approach and the interventions may prevent the cancers from occurring.

APPENDIX A – ENABLING THE USE OF LOW-LEVEL RADIATION

In this Appendix, I discuss the hurdles facing low-level radiation as an intervention and how the study of this intervention may be enabled. Let us begin by discussing the effect of low-level radiation on cancer.

The Effect of Low-Level Radiation on Cancer

You may be aware that the effect of low-level radiation on human health is presently a controversial issue with two opposite points of view prevailing in the scientific community, in spite of the subject having been studied for many decades. One point of view is that exposure to low-level radiation is beneficial, with the benefits including the reduction of cancer risk, a concept known as radiation hormesis. The other point of view is that exposure to even a very low level of radiation would increase cancer risk, a concept known as the linear no-threshold (LNT) model. Please see Appendix B for brief primers on radiation hormesis and the LNT model. Only one of these two viewpoints can be correct, because these are opposite viewpoints. Which is the correct one?

To guide the public and the governments regarding the safe use of radiation, national and international advisory bodies have been established and they periodically examine the available data and provide their recommendations. Most of the advisory bodies have supported the use of the LNT model since the 1950s (Table 9).

Table 9: Advisory bodies which do not recognize the validity of radiation hormesis but base their recommendations on the LNT model.

Advisory bodies which base their recommendations on the LNT model
National Academy of Sciences (NAS)
International Commission on Radiological Protection (ICRP)
National Council on Radiation Protection and Measurements (NCRP)
International Atomic Energy Agency (IAEA)
World Health Organization (WHO)

United Nations Scientific Committee on the Effects of Atomic Radiation (UNSCEAR)

Government regulatory agencies have accepted the recommendations of such advisory bodies and have used the LNT model as the basis for radiation protection regulations for many decades (Table 10).

Table 10. Regulatory agencies in the USA that do not recognize the validity of radiation hormesis but utilize the LNT model.

Regulatory agencies in the USA that utilize the LNT model
Environmental Protection Agency (EPA)
Nuclear Regulatory Commission (NRC)
Food and Drug Administration (FDA)

Most professional organizations have also not recognized radiation hormesis but have accepted the LNT model and utilize it for their recommendations relating to low-level radiation (Table 11).

Table 11. Professional organizations that do not recognize the validity of radiation hormesis and utilize the LNT model.

Professional organizations that utilize the LNT model
American Association of Physicists in Medicine (AAPM)
Society of Nuclear Medicine and Molecular Imaging (SNMMI)
Health Physics Society (HPS)
The Joint Commission (JC)
American College of Radiology (ACR)
The American Board of Radiology (ABR)
The Image Gently Alliance
Radiological Society of North America (RSNA)

Some of these organizations may make statements in their websites implying that they do not fully endorse the LNT model. However, their actions and the actions of their members, such as supporting dose-reduction efforts even when the radiation doses are very low, indicate that they do not recognize radiation hormesis but utilize the LNT model.

A few professional organizations and commercial enterprises, however, have recognized the validity of radiation hormesis and have recommended its study and use for improving health (Table 12).

Table 12: Professional organizations and commercial enterprises that recognize the validity of radiation hormesis.

Professional organizations that recognize the validity of radiation hormesis:
International Dose-Response Society
XLNT Foundation*
Scientists for Accurate Radiation Information (SARI)[§]
Commercial enterprises that recognize the validity of radiation hormesis:
Free-enterprise Radon Health Mine
Microsec Research & Development
Night Hawk Minerals
Sanatorium Radon, Khmelnik, Ukraine
New Energy Research Institute, Japan
Spa Dreams, Europe

*Disclosure: I am the President of the XLNT Foundation.
[§]Disclosure: I am one of the founding members of SARI.

Considering that there are professional organizations that support opposite points of view on the effect of low-level radiation on cancer, how can we decide which point of view is correct? A detailed discussion of the evidence for radiation hormesis and the LNT model may help to resolve the issue, but such a discussion would be beyond the scope of this book. Let me try to convince you that one of the preeminent advisory bodies that advocates the use of the LNT model, the NCRP, has no credibility, by discussing very briefly its latest report supporting the LNT model, the Commentary No. 27, published in 2018 [199].

This Commentary, after reviewing 29 human studies, concluded that five studies provided strong support for the LNT model. The first study they quoted is the 2017 report on the cancer incidence in the atomic bomb survivors [200]. Let us see if this publication provides strong support for the LNT model.

The abstract of this publication [200] states: "At this time, uncertainties in the shape of the dose response preclude definitive conclusions to confidently guide radiation protection policies." Such a statement indicates that the study cannot confidently determine whether cancer risk increases from the exposure to low-level radiation, because that is what would be needed to guide the radiation protection policies. Therefore, according to the publication, its data do not provide support for any model. Hence, NCRP's claim that this study provides strong support for the LNT model is clearly wrong and incredulous.

The other studies that the NCRP claimed to support the LNT model in their Commentary also do not support the LNT model, as I have explained in a couple of publications [85,201] and as discussed in another publication by Brant Ulsh [202]. NCRP has responded [203] to one of my publications, but, as you can see in my Letter to the Editor (which is at the end of a submission to ICRP: https://bit.ly/33TVWGk), they did not answer my criticisms and they unfairly refused to consider the publications supporting radiation hormesis.

It is disconcerting that the various advisory bodies, regulatory agencies and professional organizations such as listed in the Tables 9, 10, and 11 have not challenged the NCRP Commentary No. 27 for its poor quality of work, which would be obvious to even someone without much knowledge or background in the subject of radiation health effects. It is also disconcerting that these organizations have not evaluated the evidence for radiation hormesis that has been available for many decades. If they had evaluated the evidence and had recognized its validity, it would have enabled and facilitated the study of low-level radiation for cancer prevention and treatment. **Their neglect of the evidence for radiation hormesis and their implicit use of the LNT model is a major hindrance in fighting the war on cancer.**

Several debates have taken place on the health effects of low-level radiation in scientific journals, and I have participated in a couple of these debates that took place in the last few years. As you can see in these debates [204-205], the LNT model supporters have not refuted the arguments and evidence that I presented supporting radiation hormesis, whereas I have refuted the evidence they presented supporting the LNT model.

In view of this situation, I feel very confident in recommending the study of low-level radiation to prevent and treat cancer in clinical trials. However, the various advisory bodies, regulatory agencies, and professional organizations are continuing to use the LNT model. Therefore, the projected cancer risk due to low-level radiation based on the LNT model would be a major concern, making it difficult to conduct such clinical trials.

I urge all these organizations to do their due diligence, evaluate the available evidence for radiation hormesis, and recognize its validity. I also urge them to reject the LNT model, based on such evidence. It is also important that these organizations support the change in the radiation safety regulations so that they are based on radiation hormesis rather than the invalid LNT model. Such a change would facilitate the study of low-level radiation for treating and preventing cancer as well as many currently intractable diseases such as Alzheimer's disease for which the current approaches have failed repeatedly [206] and animal studies indicate that low-level radiation may be helpful in controlling the disease [207].

Once these organizations evaluate the evidence and the reasoning for radiation hormesis, accept radiation hormesis, and reject the LNT model, the use of low-level radiation would be possible as an intervention in cancer prevention clinical trials. I urge these organizations to do this evaluation promptly in the interest of public health.

Considering that the scientific and medical community has been using the LNT model for many decades, it is quite likely that you would have concerns about using low-level radiation for cancer prevention and treatment in clinical trials. To allay such concerns, I wish to bring to your attention the similarities between low-level radiation and exercise.

Both low-level radiation [208] and exercise [209] cause DNA damage and mutations in the short-term. However, when the data are examined after several months, reduced DNA damage and mutations have been observed following continuous exposure to low-level radiation [161] and regular exercise [158]. Both exercise [210] and low-level radiation [211] have led to slowing down of the tumor growth in animal studies. Both exercise [75] and low-level radiation [185] have resulted in reduced cancer mortality in humans. Both exercise [212] and low-level radiation [174] have led to improved survival for cancer patients. The recognition of such similarities between exercise and low-level radiation and the knowledge that exercise has a cancer preventive and therapeutic effect may help to allay the concerns that you may have regarding the exposure to low-level radiation.

Another way in which I can allay the concerns regarding low-level radiation is to show a few examples of reduction of cancer in the people who have been exposed to low-level radiation:

- During 1957-1981, many civilian workers overhauled and repaired nuclear-propelled US Navy ships and submarines. Among these workers, the radiation workers had exposure to low-level radiation, and the other workers (non-radiation workers) had no exposure to low-level radiation. The cancer mortality rates in the radiation workers and non-radiation workers were compiled and reported in 2005 [185]. The cancer mortality rate of the radiation workers was found to be lower by 15% (95% CI: 9-21%) when compared to the cancer mortality rate of the non-radiation workers.

- In 1982, several Co-60 sources were accidentally recycled by the steel scrap industry in northern Taiwan and resulted in contaminated steel products that were used to construct many apartment buildings. The residents of the apartment buildings received exposure to low-level radiation due to the contaminated steel in the buildings for many years. When the cancer rates in the residents of these apartment buildings were compared with an equivalent Taiwanese population, the cancer rate of the residents (who were exposed to low-level radiation) was found to be lower by 16% (95% CI: 5-26%) [178].

- The cancer mortality rate of British radiologists who entered into service during 1955-1979 (who were exposed to low-level radiation) was studied and was found to be lower by 29% (95% CI: 4-54%) when compared to the cancer rate of other physicians who were not exposed to such radiation [213].

- Patients with non-Hodgkin's Lymphoma, who were treated with repeated exposures of the whole body to low-level radiation over five weeks, had better survival than equivalent patients treated with chemotherapy, indicating that low-level radiation had a cancer therapeutic effect and not a carcinogenic effect [174].

These examples clearly show the reduction of cancer following exposure to low-level radiation, consistent with radiation hormesis. You may ask, why did the advisory bodies conclude that low levels of radiation would increase cancer risk? Is their conclusion valid? They passed such a conclusion by ignoring the data from exposure to low-level radiation such as I have mentioned above, but instead linearly extrapolating the cancer risk from the exposure to high-level radiation, using the LNT model. Though such an extrapolation has been the standard practice in the scientific community for many decades, an analogy would show that it is not a reasonable method for calculating the health effects of low-level radiation.

Would it make sense to estimate the effect of taking one caplet of medicine by studying the effect of taking 400, 200, and 100 caplets at a time and extrapolating the effects down to 1 caplet? Obviously, such an extrapolation would not make any sense. Similarly, the LNT model, which uses such an extrapolation, does not make any sense. Therefore, I would suggest that you reject the LNT model even though all the organizations listed in the above Tables 9, 10, and 11 have supported its use for many decades. You should feel confident in making use of low-level radiation for preventing and treating diseases including cancer, by participating in clinical trials or based on the advice of the organizations listed in Table 4 which recommend the use of low-level radiation for treating and preventing diseases.

Since the advisory bodies such as listed in Table 9 have supported the LNT model for many decades, it would be difficult for them to discard it and accept the opposite concept of radiation hormesis. Therefore, my recommendation is that a government committee should organize a scientific debate on radiation hormesis and it should ask the advisory bodies to refute the concept of radiation hormesis and the evidence supporting it. **If they are unable to refute radiation hormesis in such a debate, the LNT model should be declared as being invalid, and the current advisory bodies, since they have supported the LNT model while ignoring the evidence for radiation hormesis for many decades, should be defunded and disbanded.** They should be replaced by new advisory bodies which do not have the legacy of support for the LNT model and are able to recommend the use of radiation hormesis in clinical trials based on an unbiased evaluation of the evidence.

The use of the LNT model has resulted in considerable amount of harm to the society. A discussion group called Scientists for Accurate Radiation Information (SARI) was formed in 2013 to reduce and eliminate the harm caused by the misunderstanding of the health effects of low-level radiation. For full disclosure, I am one of the founding members of SARI. In this group, we have regular discussions of the health effects of low-level radiation. We also have discussions on how to reduce and eliminate the harm caused by the use of the LNT model.

An organization called the XLNT Foundation was formed a few years ago whose mission is to campaign for eliminating the use of the LNT model in order to improve human health. As a matter of full disclosure, I am the President of the XLNT Foundation. For a description of the harm caused by the use of the LNT model, please visit the XLNT Foundation website: https://www.x-lnt.org/.

The current use of the LNT model is supported by a huge infrastructure consisting of the advisory bodies, regulatory agencies, and professional organizations such as listed in the Tables 9, 10, and 11. These organizations have supported the LNT model for a long time in spite of the available evidence for radiation hormesis. Therefore, we cannot expect that these organizations would change their stance regarding the LNT model on their own. A large amount of public pressure may be needed to make them recognize radiation hormesis and reject the LNT model.

If you appreciate the importance of rejecting the LNT model for improving public health, I would suggest that you take one or more of the following steps:

1. Express your support for discarding the LNT model by answering the survey at the book website: https://bit.ly/2E1JHxj. A large public expression of support would be necessary to reform the advisory bodies and enable the use of low-level radiation in cancer prevention clinical trials.

2. Inform your friends and colleagues about the importance of discarding the LNT model through email, social media, etc. If more people become aware of the harm caused by the use of the LNT model and express their disapproval, there would be a better chance that the various organizations which presently support the LNT model would feel the pressure and correct their stance.

3. Visit the XLNT Foundation website and support its work with your comments, suggestions, donations, and by volunteering.

In summary, the use of low-level radiation as an immune boosting intervention for preventing and treating cancer in clinical trials of the I^4R approach would be possible if concerted efforts are made by a large number of interested people to defeat the dominance of the LNT model. I wish to thank you, the readers of the book, for playing your part in enabling this and contributing to reducing the cancer risk in the public and improving the outcomes for cancer patients.

APPENDIX B – RADIATION HORMESIS AND THE LNT MODEL

A Brief Primer on Radiation Hormesis

1. Exposure to low-level radiation causes some DNA damage [208].
2. Even in the absence of the low-level radiation, DNA damage does occur due to natural causes. This damage is much more than the damage due to low-level radiation [214].
3. Our body responds to the additional DNA damage due to low-level radiation by increasing the defenses such as antioxidants and DNA repair enzymes [159]. These elevated defenses last for some time.
4. The elevated defenses not only repair the damage caused by low-level radiation but also repair and prevent some of the damage that would have occurred due to natural causes.
5. The net result is that there would be reduced DNA damage and mutations following the exposure to low-level radiation, in comparison to having no additional radiation exposure [161].
6. The primary reason for the development of cancer is not cancerous mutations. Almost all of us have cancerous or pre-cancerous mutations within us [25] but only a small percentage of us have cancer at any one time.
7. The primary reason for the development of cancer is the weakening or suppression of the immune system [36]. There is plenty of data showing that when the immune system is weakened, cancer risk increases, and when the immune system is boosted, cancer risk decreases (See Chapter 2).
8. Exposure to low-level radiation causes some DNA damage [208]. The damaged cells release compounds that activate natural killer cells [215]. Other aspects of the immune system are also enhanced with the exposure to low-level radiation [216].

9. Natural killer cells and other aspects of the boosted immune system would eliminate cancer cells and so there would be fewer cancers following the exposure to low-level radiation [85].

A Brief Primer on the LNT Model

1. Even a single ray of ionizing radiation can cause DNA damage which can result in mutations [217].
2. DNA damage increases linearly with the amount of radiation exposure [208].
3. Increased mutations due to the increased DNA damage mean increased cancers, based on the mutation model of cancer [13].

Note: This reasoning for the LNT model is obviously wrong because it omits consideration of the protective biological responses and is therefore an incomplete consideration of the biological effects of the exposure to low-level radiation. The reasoning is also wrong because it pays no attention to the stimulatory effect of low-level radiation on the immune system which plays a major role in preventing cancers.

APPENDIX C – FREQUENTLY ASKED QUESTIONS

Here are some frequently asked questions regarding the book and its contents:

- Why did I write this book? The lack of major progress in the war on cancer in spite of many advances in the field indicates that a better approach may be advisable. This book presents what I consider to be a better approach to cancer.

- How important are the mutations for the development of cancer? Mutations are necessary but are not sufficient for the development of cancer. As evidence, almost all of us have cancerous or pre-cancerous mutations (covert cancers) in our body but only a small percentage of us have cancer.

- Why don't these covert cancers become real cancers? The immune system is very strong and is able to eliminate them or keep them under control.

- How do we know that the immune system is very important for preventing cancer? When the immune system is suppressed in young individuals, e.g. in young organ-transplant recipients and young AIDS patients, cancer risk increases by a factor of 40-50. Also, many studies have shown that when the immune system is enhanced, cancer risk decreases and vice versa, suggesting that weakening or suppression of the immune system is an extremely important reason, and maybe even the primary reason why cancer develops.

- How can we prevent and treat cancer? Based on the hypothesis that cancer develops primarily due to the weakening or suppression of the immune system, we can prevent and treat cancer by boosting the immune system.

- How do we boost the immune system? There are indeed many different ways of boosting the immune system (See Table 3). The immune system has many components, and different methods of boosting the immune system would enhance different components of the immune system.

- Why should we use multiple methods to boost the immune system, to prevent and treat cancer? Cancer likely occurs when the efficiencies of some immune system components decline below certain critical levels. If we boost these critical components so that they stay above the critical levels, we can possibly prevent the cancer from occurring and treat the cancer that has begun to grow. If we use only a few interventions, they may not boost the critical components and so cancer may continue to grow. If we use many different interventions, there is a better chance that the critical components would be enhanced above the critical levels, enabling the control of the cancer.

- Why should we individualize the interventions? Whereas many interventions (Table 4) can be utilized to boost the immune system, all the methods would not be applicable or acceptable to everyone, and so the interventions would need to be individualized based on the person's circumstances and preferences. The approach is known as "Individualized Interventions to Improve the Immune Response", or the I^4R approach.

- What are the main advantages of the I^4R approach? Almost all of the interventions do not have any adverse side effects. In fact, many of them have beneficial side effects. Also, many of the interventions are already known to have a cancer preventive and/or therapeutic effect.

- How can we screen for cancer? Those who have the weakest immune system response would be the ones most likely to develop cancer. Therefore, the immune system response can be measured periodically in the wide population, and those with the weakest immune system response can be identified. Immune boosting interventions can be recommended for these individuals to prevent the development of cancer.

- What are the benefits of the traditional cancer screening programs? The diagnosis of cancer from the traditional cancer screening programs can provide a useful warning sign which can motivate the individuals to take actions to boost the immune system using the I^4R approach. This may eliminate not only the detected cancers but also the cancer cells that may be lurking in other parts of the body. The interventions may also improve the health of the individuals in other ways.

- Would the I^{4}R approach give better results than the current treatments for cancer patients? Clinical trials are needed to determine this.

- What actions are needed to fully utilize the I^{4}R approach? One of the promising interventions, low-level radiation, has not been studied systematically due to the unjustified decisions of the advisory bodies supporting the LNT model. We need to reform these advisory bodies so that they perform their duties with due diligence. Thereafter, if the advisory bodies confirm that radiation hormesis is valid and the LNT model is invalid, we can start utilizing low-level radiation as an immune boosting intervention in the clinical trials of cancer prevention and treatment.

- Can we use the I^{4}R approach right now for treating and preventing cancer? No. we need to establish the validity of the approach in clinical trials. If the clinical trials establish that the I^{4}R approach is effective in preventing and treating cancer, and the medical community accepts the approach, only then we should use the I^{4}R approach for cancer prevention and treatment. **Until then, the current approach should continue to be used for preventing and treating cancer.** The I^{4}R approach may be used only under the supervision of a health-care professional as part of a clinical trial, or based on the recommendations of health-related websites such as listed in Table 4.

GLOSSARY

Age-adjusted mortality rate - A calculated mortality rate that accounts for the age distribution of the population.

AIDS - Acquired immunodeficiency syndrome.

Bariatric - Related to weight reduction.

Calorie restriction - Reduction of food intake, e.g., by 30%.

Cancer - A tumor that grows without control.

Circadian disruption - Disturbance of the 24-hour sleep-wake cycle.

Covert cancers - Cancer cells or pre-cancerous cells in the body that do not grow and develop into a tumor.

CT - Computed tomography.

DNA - Deoxyribonucleic acid. DNA is present in cells and carries genetic information.

Driver gene mutations - Mutations that help increase the growth rates of cells.

Early-stage cancer - Cancer that is early in its growth and is limited to only one area.

Forest bathing trips - Leisurely trips to the wilderness.

Hyperthermia - Elevation of body temperature.

I^4R - Individualized Interventions to Improve the Immune Response.

Late-stage cancer - Cancer that has spread from its initial location to a different part or to different parts of the body.

LNT model - The Linear No-Threshold Model. A model for estimating the cancer risk due radiation. According to this model, even the smallest amount of radiation (because there is no threshold) increases cancer risk, and as radiation dose increases, cancer risk increases linearly.

Lymphocyte - A type of white blood cell.

Lymphoma - A type of cancer that occurs in lymphocytes.

Natural killer cell - A type of white blood cell.

PET - Positron emission tomography.

Pre-leukemic cells - A precursor to leukemias.

PSA test - Prostate-specific antigen test. This is a blood test mainly used to screen for prostate cancer. PSA level is often elevated in men with prostate cancer.

Radiation hormesis - The concept that low levels of ionizing radiation are beneficial, with the beneficial effects including the reduction of cancer risk.

SMR - Standardized Mortality Ratio, i.e., the ratio of the number of observed deaths to the number of expected deaths.

Ultraviolet blood irradiation - Exposure of blood to ultraviolet light.

Xeroderma pigmentosum - A very rare skin disorder in which a person is highly sensitive to sunlight.

BIBLIOGRAPHY

1. Vrinten, C., van Jaarsveld, C. H., Waller, J., von Wagner, C. & Wardle, J. The structure and demographic correlates of cancer fear. *BMC Cancer* **14**, 597, 2014.
https://www.ncbi.nlm.nih.gov/pubmed/25129323

2. Culliton, B. J. National cancer act: deciding on people, policies, and plans. *Science* **176**, 386-390, 1972.
https://www.ncbi.nlm.nih.gov/pubmed/17777715

3. Eckhouse, S., Lewison, G. & Sullivan, R. Trends in the global funding and activity of cancer research. *Mol Oncol* **2**, 20-32, 2008.
https://www.ncbi.nlm.nih.gov/pubmed/19383326

4. Hanahan, D. & Weinberg, R. A. The hallmarks of cancer. *Cell* **100**, 57-70, 2000.
http://www.ncbi.nlm.nih.gov/pubmed/10647931

5. Hanahan, D. & Weinberg, R. A. Hallmarks of cancer: the next generation. *Cell* **144**, 646-674, 2011.
http://www.ncbi.nlm.nih.gov/pubmed/21376230

6. Petrelli, N. J. *et al.* Clinical Cancer Advances 2009: major research advances in cancer treatment, prevention, and screening--a report from the American Society of Clinical Oncology. *J Clin Oncol* **27**, 6052-6069, 2009.
https://www.ncbi.nlm.nih.gov/pubmed/19901123

7. Heymach, J. *et al.* Clinical Cancer Advances 2018: Annual Report on Progress Against Cancer From the American Society of Clinical Oncology. *J Clin Oncol* **36**, 1020-1044, 2018.
https://www.ncbi.nlm.nih.gov/pubmed/29380678

8. Faguet, G. B. *The war on cancer : an anatomy of failure, a blueprint for the future.* (Springer, 2008).
https://www.springer.com/us/book/9781402036187

9. Goldstein, I., Madar, S. & Rotter, V. Cancer research, a field on the verge of a paradigm shift? *Trends Mol Med* **18**, 299-303, 2012.
https://www.ncbi.nlm.nih.gov/pubmed/22609171

10. Xu, J., Murphy, S. L., Kochanek, K. D., Bastian, B. & Arias, E. Deaths: Final Data for 2016. *Natl Vital Stat Rep* **67**, 1-76, 2018.
https://www.ncbi.nlm.nih.gov/pubmed/30248015

11. Weir, H. K. *et al.* Heart Disease and Cancer Deaths - Trends and Projections in the United States, 1969-2020. *Prev Chronic Dis* **13**, E157, 2016.
    http://www.ncbi.nlm.nih.gov/pubmed/27854420

12. Pereira Cabral, B., da Graça Derengowski Fonseca, M. & Batista Mota, F. What is the future of cancer care? A technology foresight assessment of experts' expectations. *Economics of Innovation and New Technology*, 1-18, 2018.
    https://doi.org/10.1080/10438599.2018.1549788

13. Nordling, C. O. A new theory on cancer-inducing mechanism. *Br J Cancer* **7**, 68-72, 1953.
    http://www.ncbi.nlm.nih.gov/pubmed/13051507

14. Tomasetti, C., Li, L. & Vogelstein, B. Stem cell divisions, somatic mutations, cancer etiology, and cancer prevention. *Science* **355**, 1330-1334, 2017.
    http://www.ncbi.nlm.nih.gov/pubmed/28336671

15. Wu, S., Powers, S., Zhu, W. & Hannun, Y. A. Substantial contribution of extrinsic risk factors to cancer development. *Nature* **529**, 43-47, 2016.
    http://www.ncbi.nlm.nih.gov/pubmed/26675728

16. Martincorena, I. *et al.* Somatic mutant clones colonize the human esophagus with age. *Science* **362**, 911-917, 2018.
    https://www.ncbi.nlm.nih.gov/pubmed/30337457

17. Martincorena, I. *et al.* High burden and pervasive positive selection of somatic mutations in normal human skin. *Science* **348**, 880-886, 2015.
    http://www.ncbi.nlm.nih.gov/pubmed/25999502

18. DeGregori, J. Challenging the axiom: does the occurrence of oncogenic mutations truly limit cancer development with age? *Oncogene* **32**, 1869-1875, 2013.
    http://www.ncbi.nlm.nih.gov/pubmed/22751134

19. Thakkar, J. P., McCarthy, B. J. & Villano, J. L. Age-specific cancer incidence rates increase through the oldest age groups. *Am J Med Sci* **348**, 65-70, 2014.
    https://www.ncbi.nlm.nih.gov/pubmed/24805784

20. Norris, P. G. *et al.* Immune function, mutant frequency, and cancer risk in the DNA repair defective genodermatoses xeroderma pigmentosum, Cockayne's syndrome, and trichothiodystrophy. *J Invest Dermatol* **94**, 94-100, 1990.
    https://www.ncbi.nlm.nih.gov/pubmed/2295840

21. Bell, K. J., Del Mar, C., Wright, G., Dickinson, J. & Glasziou, P. Prevalence of incidental prostate cancer: A systematic review of autopsy studies. *Int J Cancer* **137**, 1749-1757, 2015. https://www.ncbi.nlm.nih.gov/pubmed/25821151

22. Thomas, E. T. *et al.* Prevalence of incidental breast cancer and precursor lesions in autopsy studies: a systematic review and meta-analysis. *BMC Cancer* **17**, 808, 2017. https://www.ncbi.nlm.nih.gov/pubmed/29197354

23. Mindrup, S. R., Pierre, J. S., Dahmoush, L. & Konety, B. R. The prevalence of renal cell carcinoma diagnosed at autopsy. *BJU International* **95**, 31-33, 2005. https://www.ncbi.nlm.nih.gov/pubmed/15638891

24. Matsuda, Y. *et al.* Clinicopathological Features of 15 Occult and 178 Clinical Pancreatic Ductal Adenocarcinomas in 8339 Autopsied Elderly Patients. *Pancreas* **45**, 234-240, 2016. https://www.ncbi.nlm.nih.gov/pubmed/26474426

25. Greaves, M. Does everyone develop covert cancer? *Nat Rev Cancer* **14**, 209-210, 2014. http://www.ncbi.nlm.nih.gov/pubmed/25688403

26. Mori, H. *et al.* Chromosome translocations and covert leukemic clones are generated during normal fetal development. *Proc Natl Acad Sci U S A* **99**, 8242-8247, 2002. http://www.ncbi.nlm.nih.gov/pubmed/12048236

27. Corthay, A. Does the Immune System Naturally Protect Against Cancer? *Frontiers in Immunology* **5**, 197, 2014. https://www.ncbi.nlm.nih.gov/pubmed/24860567

28. Teng, M. W., Swann, J. B., Koebel, C. M., Schreiber, R. D. & Smyth, M. J. Immune-mediated dormancy: an equilibrium with cancer. *J Leukoc Biol* **84**, 988-993, 2008. http://www.ncbi.nlm.nih.gov/pubmed/18515327

29. Allison, A. C. Tumour development following immunosuppression. *Proc R Soc Med* **63**, 1077-1080, 1970. http://www.ncbi.nlm.nih.gov/pubmed/4320709

30. Engels, E. A. *et al.* Spectrum of cancer risk among US solid organ transplant recipients. *JAMA* **306**, 1891-1901, 2011. https://www.ncbi.nlm.nih.gov/pubmed/22045767

31. Vajdic, C. M. & van Leeuwen, M. T. Cancer incidence and risk factors after solid organ transplantation. *Int J Cancer* **125**, 1747-1754, 2009.
    http://www.ncbi.nlm.nih.gov/pubmed/19444916

32. Acuna, S. A. *et al.* Cancer Mortality among recipients of solid-organ transplantation in Ontario, Canada. *JAMA Oncol* **2**, 463-469, 2016.
    http://www.ncbi.nlm.nih.gov/pubmed/26746479

33. Grulich, A. E., van Leeuwen, M. T., Falster, M. O. & Vajdic, C. M. Incidence of cancers in people with HIV/AIDS compared with immunosuppressed transplant recipients: a meta-analysis. *Lancet* **370**, 59-67, 2007.
    http://www.ncbi.nlm.nih.gov/pubmed/17617273

34. Biggar, R. J., Frisch, M. & Goedert, J. J. Risk of cancer in children with AIDS. AIDS-Cancer Match Registry Study Group. *JAMA* **284**, 205-209, 2000.
    https://www.ncbi.nlm.nih.gov/pubmed/10889594

35. Dunn, G. P., Old, L. J. & Schreiber, R. D. The three Es of cancer immunoediting. *Annu Rev Immunol* **22**, 329-360, 2004.
    http://www.ncbi.nlm.nih.gov/pubmed/15032581

36. Doss, M. Changing the Paradigm of Cancer Screening, Prevention, and Treatment. *Dose Response* **14**, 1559325816680539, 2016.
    http://www.ncbi.nlm.nih.gov/pubmed/27928220

37. Lewis, V. M., Twomey, J. J., Bealmear, P., Goldstein, G. & Good, R. A. Age, thymic involution, and circulating thymic hormone activity. *J Clin Endocrinol Metab* **47**, 145-150, 1978.
    https://www.ncbi.nlm.nih.gov/pubmed/263654

38. Hazeldine, J., Hampson, P. & Lord, J. M. Reduced release and binding of perforin at the immunological synapse underlies the age-related decline in natural killer cell cytotoxicity. *Aging Cell* **11**, 751-759, 2012.
    https://www.ncbi.nlm.nih.gov/pubmed/22642232

39. Kubota, K. *et al.* [Changes in the blood cell counts with aging]. *Nihon Ronen Igakkai Zasshi* **28**, 509-514, 1991.
    https://www.ncbi.nlm.nih.gov/pubmed/1942631

40. Levin, M. J. Immune senescence and vaccines to prevent herpes zoster in older persons. *Curr Opin Immunol* **24**, 494-500, 2012.
    http://www.ncbi.nlm.nih.gov/pubmed/22857823

41. Palmer, S., Albergante, L., Blackburn, C. C. & Newman, T. J. Thymic involution and rising disease incidence with age. *Proc Natl Acad Sci U S A* **115**, 1883-1888, 2018. https://www.ncbi.nlm.nih.gov/pubmed/29432166

42. Moolgavkar, S. H. & Knudson, A. G., Jr. Mutation and cancer: a model for human carcinogenesis. *J Natl Cancer Inst* **66**, 1037-1052, 1981. https://www.ncbi.nlm.nih.gov/pubmed/6941039

43. O'Bryan, M. K. *et al.* Cytokine profiles in the testes of rats treated with lipopolysaccharide reveal localized suppression of inflammatory responses. *Am J Physiol Regul Integr Comp Physiol* **288**, R1744-1755, 2005. https://www.ncbi.nlm.nih.gov/pubmed/15661966

44. Martin, J. A., Hamilton, B. E., Osterman, M. J., Driscoll, A. K. & Mathews, T. J. Births: Final Data for 2015. *Natl Vital Stat Rep* **66**, 1, 2017. http://www.ncbi.nlm.nih.gov/pubmed/28135188

45. Brenner, D. R., Heer, E., Ruan, Y. & Peters, C. E. The rising incidence of testicular cancer among young men in Canada, data from 1971–2015. *Cancer Epidemiology* **58**, 175-177, 2019. https://www.ncbi.nlm.nih.gov/pubmed/30616087

46. Harding, C., Pompei, F. & Wilson, R. Peak and decline in cancer incidence, mortality, and prevalence at old ages. *Cancer* **118**, 1371-1386, 2012. https://www.ncbi.nlm.nih.gov/pubmed/21953606

47. Roberts-Thomson, I. C., Whittingham, S., Youngchaiyud, U. & Mackay, I. R. Ageing, immune response, and mortality. *Lancet* **2**, 368-370, 1974. https://www.ncbi.nlm.nih.gov/pubmed/4136513

48. Jung, Y. S. *et al.* Physical Inactivity and Unhealthy Metabolic Status Are Associated with Decreased Natural Killer Cell Activity. *Yonsei Med J* **59**, 554-562, 2018. https://www.ncbi.nlm.nih.gov/pubmed/29749139

49. Patel, A. V., Maliniak, M. L., Rees-Punia, E., Matthews, C. E. & Gapstur, S. M. Prolonged Leisure Time Spent Sitting in Relation to Cause-Specific Mortality in a Large US Cohort. *Am J Epidemiol* **187**, 2151-2158, 2018. https://www.ncbi.nlm.nih.gov/pubmed/29947736

50. Stampfli, M. R. & Anderson, G. P. How cigarette smoke skews immune responses to promote infection, lung disease and cancer. *Nat Rev Immunol* **9**, 377-384, 2009.
    https://www.ncbi.nlm.nih.gov/pubmed/19330016

51. Molina, P. E., Happel, K. I., Zhang, P., Kolls, J. K. & Nelson, S. Focus on: Alcohol and the immune system. *Alcohol Res Health* **33**, 97-108, 2010.
    http://www.ncbi.nlm.nih.gov/pubmed/23579940

52. Nelson, D. E. *et al.* Alcohol-attributable cancer deaths and years of potential life lost in the United States. *Am J Public Health* **103**, 641-648, 2013.
    http://www.ncbi.nlm.nih.gov/pubmed/23409916

53. Bedrosian, T. A., Fonken, L. K., Walton, J. C. & Nelson, R. J. Chronic exposure to dim light at night suppresses immune responses in Siberian hamsters. *Biology Letters* **7**, 468-471, 2011.
    https://www.ncbi.nlm.nih.gov/pubmed/21270021

54. Hurley, S. *et al.* Light at night and breast cancer risk among California teachers. *Epidemiology* **25**, 697-706, 2014.
    http://www.ncbi.nlm.nih.gov/pubmed/25061924

55. Nobis, C. C., Kiessling, S., Labrecque, N. & Cermakian, N. Circadian Clocks and Immune Functions in *Biological Timekeeping: Clocks, Rhythms and Behaviour* (ed Vinod Kumar) 459-480 (Springer India, 2017).
    https://doi.org/10.1007/978-81-322-3688-7_22

56. Schernhammer, E. S. *et al.* Rotating night shifts and risk of breast cancer in women participating in the nurses' health study. *J Natl Cancer Inst* **93**, 1563-1568, 2001.
    http://www.ncbi.nlm.nih.gov/pubmed/11604480

57. Lennard, T. W. *et al.* The influence of surgical operations on components of the human immune system. *Br J Surg* **72**, 771-776, 1985.
    https://www.ncbi.nlm.nih.gov/pubmed/2412626

58. Caygill, C. P., Hill, M. J., Hall, C. N., Kirkham, J. S. & Northfield, T. C. Increased risk of cancer at multiple sites after gastric surgery for peptic ulcer. *Gut* **28**, 924-928, 1987.
    https://www.ncbi.nlm.nih.gov/pubmed/3666558

59. Muller, A. J. *et al.* Chronic inflammation that facilitates tumor progression creates local immune suppression by inducing

indoleamine 2,3 dioxygenase. *Proc Natl Acad Sci U S A* **105**, 17073-17078, 2008.
https://www.ncbi.nlm.nih.gov/pubmed/18952840

60. Jess, T., Rungoe, C. & Peyrin-Biroulet, L. Risk of colorectal cancer in patients with ulcerative colitis: a meta-analysis of population-based cohort studies. *Clin Gastroenterol Hepatol* **10**, 639-645, 2012.
https://www.ncbi.nlm.nih.gov/pubmed/22289873

61. Pinho, A. V., Chantrill, L. & Rooman, I. Chronic pancreatitis: a path to pancreatic cancer. *Cancer Lett* **345**, 203-209, 2014.
https://www.ncbi.nlm.nih.gov/pubmed/23981573

62. Sipponen, P. & Marshall, B. J. Gastritis and gastric cancer. Western countries. *Gastroenterol Clin North Am* **29**, 579-592, v-vi, 2000.
https://www.ncbi.nlm.nih.gov/pubmed/11030074

63. El-Serag, H. B. Epidemiology of viral hepatitis and hepatocellular carcinoma. *Gastroenterology* **142**, 1264-1273 e1261, 2012.
https://www.ncbi.nlm.nih.gov/pubmed/22537432

64. Matsuzaki, H. *et al.* Asbestos-Induced Cellular and Molecular Alteration of Immunocompetent Cells and Their Relationship with Chronic Inflammation and Carcinogenesis. *J Biomed Biotechnol* **2012**, Article ID 492608, 492609 pages,, 2012.
https://www.ncbi.nlm.nih.gov/pubmed/22500091

65. Kusters, M. A., Verstegen, R. H., Gemen, E. F. & de Vries, E. Intrinsic defect of the immune system in children with Down syndrome: a review. *Clin Exp Immunol* **156**, 189-193, 2009.
https://www.ncbi.nlm.nih.gov/pubmed/19250275

66. Miller, R. W. Neoplasia and Down's Syndrome. *Annals of the New York Academy of Sciences* **171**, 637-644, 1970.

https://nyaspubs.onlinelibrary.wiley.com/doi/abs/10.1111/j.1749-6632.1970.tb39373.x

67. Shu, X.-O. *et al.* Parental Alcohol Consumption, Cigarette Smoking, and Risk of Infant Leukemia: a Childrens Cancer Group Study. *JNCI: Journal of the National Cancer Institute* **88**, 24-31, 1996.
https://www.ncbi.nlm.nih.gov/pubmed/8847721

68. Zhang, Z. & Wang, C. Immune status of children with obstructive sleep apnea/hypopnea syndrome. *Pak J Med Sci* **33**, 195-199, 2017.

https://www.ncbi.nlm.nih.gov/pubmed/28367199
69. Campos-Rodriguez, F. *et al*. Association between obstructive sleep apnea and cancer incidence in a large multicenter Spanish cohort. *Am J Respir Crit Care Med* **187**, 99-105, 2013. https://www.ncbi.nlm.nih.gov/pubmed/23155146
70. Liu, S. Z. Nonlinear dose-response relationship in the immune system following exposure to ionizing radiation: mechanisms and implications. *Nonlinearity Biol Toxicol Med* **1**, 71-92, 2003. http://www.ncbi.nlm.nih.gov/pubmed/19330113
71. Ozasa, K. *et al*. Studies of the mortality of atomic bomb survivors, Report 14, 1950-2003: an overview of cancer and noncancer diseases. *Radiat Res* **177**, 229-243, 2012. https://www.ncbi.nlm.nih.gov/pubmed/22171960
72. Johansson, S. G. O. The discovery of IgE. *J Allergy Clin Immunol* **137**, 1671-1673, 2016. https://www.ncbi.nlm.nih.gov/pubmed/27264002
73. Wang, H. & Diepgen, T. L. Is atopy a protective or a risk factor for cancer? A review of epidemiological studies. *Allergy* **60**, 1098-1111, 2005. http://www.ncbi.nlm.nih.gov/pubmed/16076292
74. Woods, J. A. *et al*. Cardiovascular exercise training extends influenza vaccine seroprotection in sedentary older adults: the immune function intervention trial. *J Am Geriatr Soc* **57**, 2183-2191, 2009. http://www.ncbi.nlm.nih.gov/pubmed/20121985
75. Orsini, N., Mantzoros, C. S. & Wolk, A. Association of physical activity with cancer incidence, mortality, and survival: a population-based study of men. *Br J Cancer* **98**, 1864-1869, 2008. http://www.ncbi.nlm.nih.gov/pubmed/18506190
76. Evans, S. S., Repasky, E. A. & Fisher, D. T. Fever and the thermal regulation of immunity: the immune system feels the heat. *Nat Rev Immunol* **15**, 335-349, 2015. https://www.ncbi.nlm.nih.gov/pubmed/25976513
77. Kleef, R., Jonas, W. B., Knogler, W. & Stenzinger, W. Fever, cancer incidence and spontaneous remissions. *Neuroimmunomodulation* **9**, 55-64, 2001. http://www.ncbi.nlm.nih.gov/pubmed/11549887

78. Wald, E. R., Dashefsky, B., Byers, C., Guerra, N. & Taylor, F. Frequency and severity of infections in day care. *J Pediatr* **112**, 540-546, 1988.
https://www.ncbi.nlm.nih.gov/pubmed/3351677

79. Rudant, J. *et al.* Childhood acute lymphoblastic leukemia and indicators of early immune stimulation: a childhood leukemia international consortium study. *Am J Epidemiol* **181**, 549-562, 2015.
http://www.ncbi.nlm.nih.gov/pubmed/25731888

80. Bernstein, E. *et al.* Immune response to influenza vaccination in a large healthy elderly population. *Vaccine* **17**, 82-94, 1999.
http://www.ncbi.nlm.nih.gov/pubmed/10078611

81. Wang, C. S., Wang, S. T., Lai, C. T., Lin, L. J. & Chou, P. Impact of influenza vaccination on major cause-specific mortality. *Vaccine* **25**, 1196-1203, 2007.
http://www.ncbi.nlm.nih.gov/pubmed/17097773

82. Moulin, C. M., Rizzo, L. V. & Halpern, A. Effect of surgery-induced weight loss on immune function. *Expert Rev Gastroenterol Hepatol* **2**, 617-619, 2008.
https://www.ncbi.nlm.nih.gov/pubmed/19072337

83. Schauer, D. P. *et al.* Bariatric Surgery and the Risk of Cancer in a Large Multisite Cohort. *Ann Surg*, 2017.
https://www.ncbi.nlm.nih.gov/pubmed/28938270

84. Yang, G. *et al.* Low-dose ionizing radiation induces direct activation of natural killer cells and provides a novel approach for adoptive cellular immunotherapy. *Cancer biotherapy & radiopharmaceuticals* **29**, 428-434, 2014.
http://www.ncbi.nlm.nih.gov/pubmed/25402754

85. Doss, M. Are We Approaching the End of the Linear No-Threshold Era? *J Nucl Med* **59**, 1786-1793, 2018.
https://www.ncbi.nlm.nih.gov/pubmed/30262515

86. Turfkruyer, M. & Verhasselt, V. Breast milk and its impact on maturation of the neonatal immune system. *Curr Opin Infect Dis* **28**, 199-206, 2015.
http://www.ncbi.nlm.nih.gov/pubmed/25887614

87. Amitay, E. L. & Keinan-Boker, L. Breastfeeding and childhood leukemia incidence: A meta-analysis and systematic review. *JAMA Pediatr* **169**, e151025, 2015.
http://www.ncbi.nlm.nih.gov/pubmed/26030516

88. Imai, K., Matsuyama, S., Miyake, S., Suga, K. & Nakachi, K. Natural cytotoxic activity of peripheral-blood lymphocytes and cancer incidence: an 11-year follow-up study of a general population. *Lancet* **356**, 1795-1799, 2000. https://www.ncbi.nlm.nih.gov/pubmed/11117911

89. Levy, S. M., Herberman, R. B., Lippman, M., D'Angelo, T. & Lee, J. Immunological and psychosocial predictors of disease recurrence in patients with early-stage breast cancer. *Behav Med* **17**, 67-75, 1991. https://www.ncbi.nlm.nih.gov/pubmed/1878611

90. Spiering, M. J. Primer on the Immune System. *Alcohol Res* **37**, 171-175, 2015. https://www.ncbi.nlm.nih.gov/pubmed/26695756

91. Idorn, M. & Hojman, P. Exercise-Dependent Regulation of NK Cells in Cancer Protection. *Trends Mol Med* **22**, 565-577, 2016. https://www.ncbi.nlm.nih.gov/pubmed/27262760

92. Leelarungrayub, D. *et al.* Six weeks of aerobic dance exercise improves blood oxidative stress status and increases interleukin-2 in previously sedentary women. *J Bodyw Mov Ther* **15**, 355-362, 2011. https://www.ncbi.nlm.nih.gov/pubmed/21665113

93. Nieman, D. C. *et al.* Physical activity and immune function in elderly women. *Med Sci Sports Exerc* **25**, 823-831, 1993. http://www.ncbi.nlm.nih.gov/pubmed/8350705

94. Shinkai, S. *et al.* Physical activity and immune senescence in men. *Med Sci Sports Exerc* **27**, 1516-1526, 1995. http://www.ncbi.nlm.nih.gov/pubmed/8587488

95. Yan, H. *et al.* Effect of moderate exercise on immune senescence in men. *Eur J Appl Physiol* **86**, 105-111, 2001. https://www.ncbi.nlm.nih.gov/pubmed/11822468

96. Woods, J. A. *et al.* Effects of 6 months of moderate aerobic exercise training on immune function in the elderly. *Mech Ageing Dev* **109**, 1-19, 1999. https://www.ncbi.nlm.nih.gov/pubmed/10405985

97. Fairey, A. S. *et al.* Randomized controlled trial of exercise and blood immune function in postmenopausal breast cancer survivors. *J Appl Physiol (1985)* **98**, 1534-1540, 2005. https://www.ncbi.nlm.nih.gov/pubmed/15772062

98. Kohut, M. L. *et al.* Moderate exercise improves antibody response to influenza immunization in older adults. *Vaccine* **22**, 2298-2306, 2004.
https://www.ncbi.nlm.nih.gov/pubmed/15149789

99. Pilch, W. *et al.* Effect of a single finnish sauna session on white blood cell profile and cortisol levels in athletes and non-athletes. *J Hum Kinet* **39**, 127-135, 2013.
http://www.ncbi.nlm.nih.gov/pubmed/24511348

100. Brazaitis, M. *et al.* Two strategies for response to 14 degrees C cold-water immersion: is there a difference in the response of motor, cognitive, immune and stress markers? *PLoS One* **9**, e109020, 2014.
https://www.ncbi.nlm.nih.gov/pubmed/25275647

101. Li, Q. Effect of forest bathing trips on human immune function. *Environ Health Prev Med* **15**, 9-17, 2010.
http://www.ncbi.nlm.nih.gov/pubmed/19568839

102. Mishra, K. P. & Ganju, L. Influence of high altitude exposure on the immune system: a review. *Immunol Invest* **39**, 219-234, 2010.
https://www.ncbi.nlm.nih.gov/pubmed/20380520

103. Phan, T. X., Jaruga, B., Pingle, S. C., Bandyopadhyay, B. C. & Ahern, G. P. Intrinsic Photosensitivity Enhances Motility of T Lymphocytes. *Sci Rep* **6**, 39479, 2016.
http://www.ncbi.nlm.nih.gov/pubmed/27995987

104. Lim, S. A. & Cheong, K. J. Regular Yoga Practice Improves Antioxidant Status, Immune Function, and Stress Hormone Releases in Young Healthy People: A Randomized, Double-Blind, Controlled Pilot Study. *J Altern Complement Med* **21**, 530-538, 2015.
http://www.ncbi.nlm.nih.gov/pubmed/26181573

105. Kochupillai, V. *et al.* Effect of rhythmic breathing (Sudarshan Kriya and Pranayam) on immune functions and tobacco addiction. *Ann N Y Acad Sci* **1056**, 242-252, 2005.
http://www.ncbi.nlm.nih.gov/pubmed/16387692

106. Black, D. S. & Slavich, G. M. Mindfulness meditation and the immune system: a systematic review of randomized controlled trials. *Ann N Y Acad Sci* **1373**, 13-24, 2016.
https://www.ncbi.nlm.nih.gov/pubmed/26799456

107. Bennett, M. P., Zeller, J. M., Rosenberg, L. & McCann, J. The effect of mirthful laughter on stress and natural killer cell activity. *Altern Ther Health Med* **9**, 38-45, 2003. http://www.ncbi.nlm.nih.gov/pubmed/12652882

108. Yeh, S. H., Chuang, H., Lin, L. W., Hsiao, C. Y. & Eng, H. L. Regular tai chi chuan exercise enhances functional mobility and CD4CD25 regulatory T cells. *Br J Sports Med* **40**, 239-243, 2006. https://www.ncbi.nlm.nih.gov/pubmed/16505081

109. Frączek, P., Kilian-Kita, A., Püsküllüoglu, M. & Krzemieniecki, K. Acupuncture as anticancer treatment? *Contemp Oncol (Pozn)* **20**, 453-457, 2016. https://www.ncbi.nlm.nih.gov/pubmed/28239282

110. Meliska, C. J., Stunkard, M. E., Gilbert, D. G., Jensen, R. A. & Martinko, J. M. Immune function in cigarette smokers who quit smoking for 31 days. *J Allergy Clin Immunol* **95**, 901-910, 1995. https://www.ncbi.nlm.nih.gov/pubmed/7722172

111. Ahmed, T. *et al.* Calorie restriction enhances T-cell-mediated immune response in adult overweight men and women. *J Gerontol A Biol Sci Med Sci* **64**, 1107-1113, 2009. https://www.ncbi.nlm.nih.gov/pubmed/19638417

112. Meydani, S. N. *et al.* Long-term moderate calorie restriction inhibits inflammation without impairing cell-mediated immunity: a randomized controlled trial in non-obese humans. *Aging (Albany NY)* **8**, 1416-1431, 2016. https://www.ncbi.nlm.nih.gov/pubmed/27410480

113. Faris, M. A. *et al.* Intermittent fasting during Ramadan attenuates proinflammatory cytokines and immune cells in healthy subjects. *Nutrition Research* **32**, 947-955, 2012. https://www.ncbi.nlm.nih.gov/pubmed/23244540

114. Gibson, A. *et al.* Effect of fruit and vegetable consumption on immune function in older people: a randomized controlled trial. *Am J Clin Nutr* **96**, 1429-1436, 2012. http://www.ncbi.nlm.nih.gov/pubmed/23134881

115. Aranow, C. Vitamin D and the immune system. *J Investig Med* **59**, 881-886, 2011. http://www.ncbi.nlm.nih.gov/pubmed/21527855

116. Perdigon, G., Valdez, J. C. & Rachid, M. Antitumour activity of yogurt: study of possible immune mechanisms. *J Dairy Res* **65**, 129-138, 1998.

https://www.ncbi.nlm.nih.gov/pubmed/9513059

117. Gill, H. S. & Guarner, F. Probiotics and human health: a clinical perspective. *Postgraduate Medical Journal* **80**, 516-526, 2004. https://www.ncbi.nlm.nih.gov/pubmed/15356352

118. Vanegas, S. M. *et al.* Substituting whole grains for refined grains in a 6-wk randomized trial has a modest effect on gut microbiota and immune and inflammatory markers of healthy adults. *The American Journal of Clinical Nutrition* **105**, 635-650, 2017. https://www.ncbi.nlm.nih.gov/pubmed/28179226

119. Bild, W. *et al.* Research concerning the radioprotective and immunostimulating effects of deuterium-depleted water. *Rom J Physiol* **36**, 205-218, 1999. https://www.ncbi.nlm.nih.gov/pubmed/11797936

120. Chiang, N., Bermudez, E. A., Ridker, P. M., Hurwitz, S. & Serhan, C. N. Aspirin triggers antiinflammatory 15-epi-lipoxin A4 and inhibits thromboxane in a randomized human trial. *Proc Natl Acad Sci U S A* **101**, 15178-15183, 2004. https://www.ncbi.nlm.nih.gov/pubmed/15471991

121. Gruenbacher, G. *et al.* IL-2 costimulation enables statin-mediated activation of human NK cells, preferentially through a mechanism involving CD56+ dendritic cells. *Cancer Res* **70**, 9611-9620, 2010. https://www.ncbi.nlm.nih.gov/pubmed/20947520

122. Cao, Y. *et al.* Meat intake and risk of diverticulitis among men. *Gut* **67**, 466-472, 2018. https://www.ncbi.nlm.nih.gov/pubmed/28069830

123. Viardot, A., Lord, R. V. & Samaras, K. The effects of weight loss and gastric banding on the innate and adaptive immune system in type 2 diabetes and prediabetes. *J Clin Endocrinol Metab* **95**, 2845-2850, 2010. https://www.ncbi.nlm.nih.gov/pubmed/20375213

124. Field, T. Chapter 9 - Enhancing immune function in *Massage Therapy Research* (ed Tiffany Field) 157-175 (Churchill Livingstone, 2006). https://doi.org/10.1016/B978-0-443-10201-1.50013-1

125. Ganz, F. D. Sleep and immune function. *Crit Care Nurse* **32**, e19-25, 2012. http://www.ncbi.nlm.nih.gov/pubmed/22467620

126. Nagai, M. *et al.* Effects of Fatigue on Immune Function in Nurses Performing Shift Work. *Journal of Occupational Health* **53**, 312-319, 2011.
     https://www.ncbi.nlm.nih.gov/pubmed/21778660

127. Cohen, L. *et al.* Presurgical Stress Management Improves Postoperative Immune Function in Men With Prostate Cancer Undergoing Radical Prostatectomy. *Psychosomatic Medicine* **73**, 218-225, 2011.
     https://www.ncbi.nlm.nih.gov/pubmed/21257977

128. Haake, P. *et al.* Effects of sexual arousal on lymphocyte subset circulation and cytokine production in man. *Neuroimmunomodulation* **11**, 293-298, 2004.
     https://www.ncbi.nlm.nih.gov/pubmed/15316239

129. Murray, D. R., Haselton, M. G., Fales, M. & Cole, S. W. Falling in love is associated with immune system gene regulation. *Psychoneuroendocrinology* **100**, 120-126, 2019.
     https://www.ncbi.nlm.nih.gov/pubmed/30299259

130. Hassiotou, F. *et al.* Maternal and infant infections stimulate a rapid leukocyte response in breastmilk. *Clin Transl Immunology* **2**, e3, 2013.
     https://www.ncbi.nlm.nih.gov/pubmed/25505951

131. Schapiro, J. M., Segev, Y., Rannon, L., Alkan, M. & Rager-Zisman, B. Natural killer (NK) cell response after vaccination of volunteers with killed influenza vaccine. *J Med Virol* **30**, 196-200, 1990.
     https://www.ncbi.nlm.nih.gov/pubmed/2341835

132. Pulendran, B. Learning immunology from the yellow fever vaccine: innate immunity to systems vaccinology. *Nature Reviews Immunology* **9**, 741, 2009.
     https://www.ncbi.nlm.nih.gov/pubmed/19763148

133. Majumder, P. P. Genomics of immune response to typhoid and cholera vaccines. *Philos Trans R Soc Lond B Biol Sci* **370**, 2015.
     https://www.ncbi.nlm.nih.gov/pubmed/25964454

134. Simkó, M. & Mattsson, M.-O. Extremely low frequency electromagnetic fields as effectors of cellular responses in vitro: Possible immune cell activation. *Journal of Cellular Biochemistry* **93**, 83-92, 2004.
     https://www.ncbi.nlm.nih.gov/pubmed/15352165

135. Ruhle, P. F. *et al.* Modulation of the peripheral immune system after low-dose radon spa therapy: Detailed longitudinal immune

monitoring of patients within the RAD-ON01 study. *Autoimmunity* **50**, 133-140, 2017. http://www.ncbi.nlm.nih.gov/pubmed/28263099

136. Wu, X., Hu, X. & Hamblin, M. R. Ultraviolet blood irradiation: Is it time to remember "the cure that time forgot"? *J Photochem Photobiol B* **157**, 89-96, 2016. http://www.ncbi.nlm.nih.gov/pubmed/26894849

137. Elvis, A. M. & Ekta, J. S. Ozone therapy: A clinical review. *J Nat Sci Biol Med* **2**, 66-70, 2011. https://www.ncbi.nlm.nih.gov/pubmed/22470237

138. Farjadian, S., Norouzian, M., Younesi, V., Ebrahimpour, A. & Lotfi, R. Hyperthermia increases natural killer cell cytotoxicity against SW-872 liposarcoma cell line. *Iran J Immunol* **10**, 93-102, 2013. https://www.ncbi.nlm.nih.gov/pubmed/23811548

139. Rodriguez-Miguelez, P. *et al.* Whole-body vibration improves the anti-inflammatory status in elderly subjects through toll-like receptor 2 and 4 signaling pathways. *Mechanisms of Ageing and Development* **150**, 12-19, 2015. https://www.ncbi.nlm.nih.gov/pubmed/26253933

140. Weisz, G. *et al.* Modification of in Vivo and in Vitro TNF-α, IL-1, and IL-6 Secretion by Circulating Monocytes During Hyperbaric Oxygen Treatment in Patients with Perianal Crohn's Disease. *Journal of Clinical Immunology* **17**, 154-159, 1997. https://www.ncbi.nlm.nih.gov/pubmed/9083891

141. Karbach, J. *et al.* Phase I clinical trial of mixed bacterial vaccine (Coley's toxins) in patients with NY-ESO-1 expressing cancers: immunological effects and clinical activity. *Clin Cancer Res* **18**, 5449-5459, 2012. http://www.ncbi.nlm.nih.gov/pubmed/22847809

142. Gauthier, T. W., Drews-Botsch, C., Falek, A., Coles, C. & Brown, L. A. Maternal alcohol abuse and neonatal infection. *Alcohol Clin Exp Res* **29**, 1035-1043, 2005. https://www.ncbi.nlm.nih.gov/pubmed/15976530

143. Jackson, K. M. & Nazar, A. M. Breastfeeding, the immune response, and long-term health. *J Am Osteopath Assoc* **106**, 203-207, 2006. https://www.ncbi.nlm.nih.gov/pubmed/16627775

144. Ang, J. Y. *et al.* A randomized placebo-controlled trial of massage therapy on the immune system of preterm infants. *Pediatrics* **130**, e1549-1558, 2012.
https://www.ncbi.nlm.nih.gov/pubmed/23147978

145. Bergroth, E. *et al.* Respiratory tract illnesses during the first year of life: effect of dog and cat contacts. *Pediatrics* **130**, 211-220, 2012.
https://www.ncbi.nlm.nih.gov/pubmed/22778307

146. Otto, S. *et al.* General Non-specific Morbidity is Reduced After Vaccination Within the Third Month of Life - the Greifswald Study. *Journal of Infection* **41**, 172-175, 2000.
https://www.ncbi.nlm.nih.gov/pubmed/11023764

147. Jessy, T. Immunity over inability: The spontaneous regression of cancer. *J Nat Sci Biol Med* **2**, 43-49, 2011.
https://www.ncbi.nlm.nih.gov/pubmed/22470233

148. Coley, W. B. The Treatment of Inoperable Sarcoma by Bacterial Toxins (the Mixed Toxins of the Streptococcus erysipelas and the Bacillus prodigiosus). *Proc R Soc Med* **3**, 1-48, 1910.
http://www.ncbi.nlm.nih.gov/pubmed/19974799

149. Coley, W. B. The treatment of malignant tumors by repeated inoculations of erysipelas. With a report of ten original cases. 1893. *Clin Orthop Relat Res*, 3-11, 1991.
https://www.ncbi.nlm.nih.gov/pubmed/1984929

150. Kronz, J. D., Westra, W. H. & Epstein, J. I. Mandatory second opinion surgical pathology at a large referral hospital. *Cancer* **86**, 2426-2435, 1999.
https://www.ncbi.nlm.nih.gov/pubmed/10590387

151. Payne, V. L. *et al.* Patient-Initiated Second Opinions: Systematic Review of Characteristics and Impact on Diagnosis, Treatment, and Satisfaction. *Mayo Clinic Proceedings* **89**, 687-696, 2014.
https://www.ncbi.nlm.nih.gov/pubmed/24797646

152. Connolly, R. M. *et al.* TBCRC026: Phase II Trial Correlating Standardized Uptake Value With Pathologic Complete Response to Pertuzumab and Trastuzumab in Breast Cancer. *J Clin Oncol*, JCO2018787986, 2019.
https://www.ncbi.nlm.nih.gov/pubmed/30721110

153. Fuerea, A. *et al.* Early PSA response is an independent prognostic factor in patients with metastatic castration-resistant prostate cancer treated with next-generation androgen pathway inhibitors. *European Journal of Cancer* **61**, 44-51, 2016.

https://www.ncbi.nlm.nih.gov/pubmed/27151554

154. Dowdy, S. C., Stefanek, M. & Hartmann, L. C. Surgical risk reduction: prophylactic salpingo-oophorectomy and prophylactic mastectomy. *Am J Obstet Gynecol* **191**, 1113-1123, 2004. https://www.ncbi.nlm.nih.gov/pubmed/15507929

155. Heemskerk-Gerritsen, B. A. M. *et al.* Survival after bilateral risk-reducing mastectomy in healthy BRCA1 and BRCA2 mutation carriers. *Breast Cancer Research and Treatment*, 2019. https://www.ncbi.nlm.nih.gov/pubmed/31302855

156. Pettapiece-Phillips, R., Narod, S. A. & Kotsopoulos, J. The role of body size and physical activity on the risk of breast cancer in BRCA mutation carriers. *Cancer Causes Control* **26**, 333-344, 2015. https://www.ncbi.nlm.nih.gov/pubmed/25579073

157. Kotsopoulos, J. *et al.* Changes in body weight and the risk of breast cancer in BRCA1 and BRCA2 mutation carriers. *Breast Cancer Res* **7**, R833-843, 2005. https://www.ncbi.nlm.nih.gov/pubmed/16168130

158. Soares, J. P. *et al.* Effects of combined physical exercise training on DNA damage and repair capacity: role of oxidative stress changes. *Age (Dordr)* **37**, 9799, 2015. https://www.ncbi.nlm.nih.gov/pubmed/26044257

159. Feinendegen, L. E., Pollycove, M. & Neumann, R. D. Hormesis by Low Dose Radiation Effects: Low-Dose Cancer Risk Modeling Must Recognize Up-Regulation of Protection in *Therapeutic Nuclear Medicine* (ed Richard P. Baum) (Springer, 2013). http://link.springer.com/chapter/10.1007/174_2012_686

160. Koana, T. & Tsujimura, H. A U-shaped dose-response relationship between x radiation and sex-linked recessive lethal mutation in male germ cells of Drosophila. *Radiat Res* **174**, 46-51, 2010. http://www.ncbi.nlm.nih.gov/pubmed/20681798

161. Osipov, A. N., Buleeva, G., Arkhangelskaya, E. & Klokov, D. In vivo gamma-irradiation low dose threshold for suppression of DNA double strand breaks below the spontaneous level in mouse blood and spleen cells. *Mutat Res* **756**, 141-145, 2013. http://www.ncbi.nlm.nih.gov/pubmed/23664857

162. Kakinuma, S., Yamauchi, K., Amasaki, Y., Nishimura, M. & Shimada, Y. Low-dose radiation attenuates chemical mutagenesis in vivo. *J Radiat Res* **50**, 401-405, 2009. http://www.ncbi.nlm.nih.gov/pubmed/19680009

163. Ghiassi-nejad, M., Mortazavi, S. M., Cameron, J. R., Niroomand-rad, A. & Karam, P. A. Very high background radiation areas of Ramsar, Iran: preliminary biological studies. *Health Phys* **82**, 87-93, 2002. http://www.ncbi.nlm.nih.gov/pubmed/11769138

164. Xu, J., Neale, A. V., Dailey, R. K., Eggly, S. & Schwartz, K. L. Patient perspective on watchful waiting/active surveillance for localized prostate cancer. *J Am Board Fam Med* **25**, 763-770, 2012. https://www.ncbi.nlm.nih.gov/pubmed/23136314

165. Burt, L. M., Ying, J., Poppe, M. M., Suneja, G. & Gaffney, D. K. Risk of secondary malignancies after radiation therapy for breast cancer: Comprehensive results. *Breast* **35**, 122-129, 2017. http://www.ncbi.nlm.nih.gov/pubmed/28719811

166. Swerdlow, A. J. *et al.* Second cancer risk after chemotherapy for Hodgkin's lymphoma: a collaborative British cohort study. *J Clin Oncol* **29**, 4096-4104, 2011. https://www.ncbi.nlm.nih.gov/pubmed/21969511

167. Lee, I. M., Wolin, K. Y., Freeman, S. E., Sattlemair, J. & Sesso, H. D. Physical activity and survival after cancer diagnosis in men. *J Phys Act Health* **11**, 85-90, 2014. http://www.ncbi.nlm.nih.gov/pubmed/23250326

168. Guinter, M. A., McCullough, M. L., Gapstur, S. M. & Campbell, P. T. Associations of Pre- and Postdiagnosis Diet Quality With Risk of Mortality Among Men and Women With Colorectal Cancer. *J Clin Oncol*, JCO1800714, 2018. https://www.ncbi.nlm.nih.gov/pubmed/30339519

169. Warren, G. W., Kasza, K. A., Reid, M. E., Cummings, K. M. & Marshall, J. R. Smoking at diagnosis and survival in cancer patients. *Int J Cancer* **132**, 401-410, 2013. https://www.ncbi.nlm.nih.gov/pubmed/22539012

170. Elwood, P. C. *et al.* Systematic review update of observational studies further supports aspirin role in cancer treatment: Time to share evidence and decision-making with patients? *PLoS One* **13**, e0203957, 2018. https://www.ncbi.nlm.nih.gov/pubmed/30252883

171. Giese-Davis, J. *et al.* Decrease in depression symptoms is associated with longer survival in patients with metastatic breast cancer: a secondary analysis. *Journal of clinical oncology* **29**, 413-420, 2011.
https://www.ncbi.nlm.nih.gov/pubmed/21149651

172. Ji, J., Sundquist, J. & Sundquist, K. Association between post-diagnostic use of cholera vaccine and risk of death in prostate cancer patients. *Nat Commun* **9**, 2367-2367, 2018.
https://www.ncbi.nlm.nih.gov/pubmed/29915319

173. Franckena, M. *et al.* Long-term improvement in treatment outcome after radiotherapy and hyperthermia in locoregionally advanced cervix cancer: an update of the Dutch Deep Hyperthermia Trial. *Int J Radiat Oncol Biol Phys* **70**, 1176-1182, 2008.
https://www.ncbi.nlm.nih.gov/pubmed/17881144

174. Pollycove, M. Radiobiological Basis of Low-Dose Irradiation in Prevention and Therapy of Cancer. *Dose-Response* **5**, 26-38, 2007.
http://www.ncbi.nlm.nih.gov/pubmed/18648556

175. Saito, E. *et al.* Smoking cessation and subsequent risk of cancer: A pooled analysis of eight population-based cohort studies in Japan. *Cancer Epidemiol* **51**, 98-108, 2017.
https://www.ncbi.nlm.nih.gov/pubmed/29102692

176. Hu, Y.-B., Hu, E.-D. & Fu, R.-Q. Statin Use and Cancer Incidence in Patients with Type 2 Diabetes Mellitus: A Network Meta-Analysis. *Gastroenterology Research and Practice* **2018**, 10, 2018.
https://www.ncbi.nlm.nih.gov/pubmed/30254671

177. Han, M. A. *et al.* Reduction of Red and Processed Meat Intake and Cancer Mortality and Incidence: A Systematic Review and Meta-analysis of Cohort Studies. *Annals of Internal Medicine*, [Epub ahead of print]. doi: 10.7326/M7319-0699., 2019.
https://www.ncbi.nlm.nih.gov/pubmed/31569214

178. Doss, M. Comment on '30 years follow-up and increased risks of breast cancer and leukaemia after long-term low-dose-rate radiation exposure'. *Br J Cancer* **118**, e9, 2018.
https://www.ncbi.nlm.nih.gov/pubmed/29438374

179. Orsi, L. *et al.* Living on a farm, contact with farm animals and pets, and childhood acute lymphoblastic leukemia: pooled and

meta-analyses from the Childhood Leukemia International Consortium. *Cancer Med* **7**, 2665-2681, 2018. https://www.ncbi.nlm.nih.gov/pubmed/29663688

180. Morra, M. E. *et al.* Early vaccination protects against childhood leukemia: A systematic review and meta-analysis. *Sci Rep* **7**, 15986, 2017. https://www.ncbi.nlm.nih.gov/pubmed/29167460

181. McLaughlin, J. K., Hrubsec, Z., Blot, W. J. & Fraumeni Jr., J. F. Smoking and cancer mortality among U.S. veterans: A 26-year follow-up. *International Journal of Cancer* **60**, 190-193, 1995. https://www.ncbi.nlm.nih.gov/pubmed/7829214

182. Aune, D. *et al.* Fruit and vegetable intake and the risk of cardiovascular disease, total cancer and all-cause mortality-a systematic review and dose-response meta-analysis of prospective studies. *Int J Epidemiol* **46**, 1029-1056, 2017. https://www.ncbi.nlm.nih.gov/pubmed/28338764

183. Nielsen, S. F., Nordestgaard, B. G. & Bojesen, S. E. Statin Use and Reduced Cancer-Related Mortality. *New England Journal of Medicine* **367**, 1792-1802, 2012. https://www.ncbi.nlm.nih.gov/pubmed/23134381/

184. Keum, N., Lee, D. H., Greenwood, D. C., Manson, J. E. & Giovannucci, E. Vitamin D supplementation and total cancer incidence and mortality: a meta-analysis of randomized controlled trials. *Ann Oncol* **30**, 733-743, 2019. https://www.ncbi.nlm.nih.gov/pubmed/30796437

185. Sponsler, R. & Cameron, J. R. Nuclear shipyard worker study (1980-1988): a large cohort exposed to low-dose-rate gamma radiation. *Int J Low Radiat* **1**, 463-478, 2005. http://www.inderscience.com/info/inarticle.php?artid=7915

186. Carlson, S. A., Fulton, J. E., Pratt, M., Yang, Z. & Adams, E. K. Inadequate physical activity and health care expenditures in the United States. *Prog Cardiovasc Dis* **57**, 315-323, 2015. https://www.ncbi.nlm.nih.gov/pubmed/25559060

187. Middleton, K. R., Anton, S. D. & Perri, M. G. Long-Term Adherence to Health Behavior Change. *Am J Lifestyle Med* **7**, 395-404, 2013. https://www.ncbi.nlm.nih.gov/pubmed/27547170

188. Ma, A. M. *et al.* Noncompliance with adjuvant radiation, chemotherapy, or hormonal therapy in breast cancer patients. *Am J Surg* **196**, 500-504, 2008.

https://www.ncbi.nlm.nih.gov/pubmed/18809051

189. Wallace, S. K. *et al.* Refusal of Recommended Chemotherapy for Ovarian Cancer: Risk Factors and Outcomes; a National Cancer Data Base Study. *J Natl Compr Canc Netw* **14**, 539-550, 2016. https://www.ncbi.nlm.nih.gov/pubmed/27160232

190. Joseph, K. *et al.* Outcome analysis of breast cancer patients who declined evidence-based treatment. *World J Surg Oncol* **10**, 118, 2012. https://www.ncbi.nlm.nih.gov/pubmed/22734852

191. Huang, H.-L., Kung, P.-T., Chiu, C.-F., Wang, Y.-H. & Tsai, W.-C. Factors Associated with Lung Cancer Patients Refusing Treatment and Their Survival: A National Cohort Study under a Universal Health Insurance in Taiwan. *PLOS ONE* **9**, e101731, 2014. https://www.ncbi.nlm.nih.gov/pubmed/24999633

192. Chong, C. R. & Janne, P. A. The quest to overcome resistance to EGFR-targeted therapies in cancer. *Nat Med* **19**, 1389-1400, 2013. https://www.ncbi.nlm.nih.gov/pubmed/24202392

193. Rebucci, M. & Michiels, C. Molecular aspects of cancer cell resistance to chemotherapy. *Biochem Pharmacol* **85**, 1219-1226, 2013. https://www.ncbi.nlm.nih.gov/pubmed/23435357

194. Tannock, I. F. & Hickman, J. A. Limits to Personalized Cancer Medicine. *N Engl J Med* **375**, 1289-1294, 2016. https://www.ncbi.nlm.nih.gov/pubmed/27682039

195. Chen, C. D. *et al.* Molecular determinants of resistance to antiandrogen therapy. *Nat Med* **10**, 33-39, 2004. https://www.ncbi.nlm.nih.gov/pubmed/14702632

196. Giuliano, S. & Pages, G. Mechanisms of resistance to anti-angiogenesis therapies. *Biochimie* **95**, 1110-1119, 2013. https://www.ncbi.nlm.nih.gov/pubmed/23507428

197. Seto, T., Sam, D. & Pan, M. Mechanisms of Primary and Secondary Resistance to Immune Checkpoint Inhibitors in Cancer. *Med Sci (Basel)* **7**, 2019. https://www.ncbi.nlm.nih.gov/pubmed/30678257

198. Shah, N. N. & Fry, T. J. Mechanisms of resistance to CAR T cell therapy. *Nat Rev Clin Oncol*, 2019. https://www.ncbi.nlm.nih.gov/pubmed/30837712

199. NCRP. Commentary No. 27 - Implications of recent epidemiologic studies for the linear-nonthreshold model and radiation protection. 210 (National Council on Radiation Protection and Measurements, Bethesda, MD, 2018). https://ncrponline.org/shop/commentaries/commentary-no-27-implications-of-recent-epidemiologic-studies-for-the-linear-nonthreshold-model-and-radiation-protection-2018/

200. Grant, E. J. *et al.* Solid cancer incidence among the life span study of atomic bomb survivors: 1958-2009. *Radiat Res* **187**, 513-537, 2017. http://www.ncbi.nlm.nih.gov/pubmed/28319463

201. Doss, M. Comment on 'Implications of recent epidemiologic studies for the linear nonthreshold model and radiation protection'. *Journal of Radiological Protection* **39**, 650-654, 2019. https://www.ncbi.nlm.nih.gov/pubmed/31125319

202. Ulsh, B. A. A critical evaluation of the NCRP COMMENTARY 27 endorsement of the linear no-threshold model of radiation effects. *Environ Res* **167**, 472-487, 2018. https://www.ncbi.nlm.nih.gov/pubmed/30138826

203. Shore, R. E. *et al.* Reply to Comment on 'Implications of recent epidemiologic studies for the linear nonthreshold model and radiation protection'. *Journal of Radiological Protection* **39**, 655-659, 2019. https://www.ncbi.nlm.nih.gov/pubmed/31125317

204. Doss, M. COUNTERPOINT: Should Radiation Dose From CT Scans Be a Factor in Patient Care? No. *Chest* **147**, 874-877, 2015. http://www.ncbi.nlm.nih.gov/pubmed/25846525

205. Doss, M., Little, M. P. & Orton, C. G. Point/Counterpoint: low-dose radiation is beneficial, not harmful. *Med Phys* **41**, 070601, 2014. https://www.ncbi.nlm.nih.gov/pubmed/24989368

206. Aisen, P. S. Editorial: Failure After Failure. What Next in AD Drug Development? *J Prev Alzheimers Dis* **6**, 150, 2019. https://www.ncbi.nlm.nih.gov/pubmed/31062821

207. Wei, L. C. *et al.* Low-dose radiation stimulates Wnt/beta-catenin signaling, neural stem cell proliferation and neurogenesis of the mouse hippocampus in vitro and in vivo. *Current Alzheimer Research* **9**, 278-289, 2012.

http://www.ncbi.nlm.nih.gov/pubmed/22272614

208. Vandevoorde, C. *et al.* gamma-H2AX foci as in vivo effect biomarker in children emphasize the importance to minimize x-ray doses in paediatric CT imaging. *Eur Radiol* **25**, 800-811, 2015.
http://www.ncbi.nlm.nih.gov/pubmed/25354556

209. Fogarty, M. C. *et al.* Exercise-induced lipid peroxidation: Implications for deoxyribonucleic acid damage and systemic free radical generation. *Environ Mol Mutagen* **52**, 35-42, 2011.
http://www.ncbi.nlm.nih.gov/pubmed/20839226

210. Pedersen, L. *et al.* Voluntary Running Suppresses Tumor Growth through Epinephrine- and IL-6-Dependent NK Cell Mobilization and Redistribution. *Cell Metabolism* **23**, 554-562, 2016.
https://www.ncbi.nlm.nih.gov/pubmed/26895752

211. Lemon, J. A., Phan, N. & Boreham, D. R. Multiple CT Scans Extend Lifespan by Delaying Cancer Progression in Cancer-Prone Mice. *Radiat Res* **188**, 495-504, 2017.
https://www.ncbi.nlm.nih.gov/pubmed/28741984

212. Cormie, P., Zopf, E. M., Zhang, X. & Schmitz, K. H. The Impact of Exercise on Cancer Mortality, Recurrence, and Treatment-Related Adverse Effects. *Epidemiol Rev* **39**, 71-92, 2017.
https://www.ncbi.nlm.nih.gov/pubmed/28453622

213. Berrington, A., Darby, S. C., Weiss, H. A. & Doll, R. 100 years of observation on British radiologists: mortality from cancer and other causes 1897-1997. *Br J Radiol* **74**, 507-519, 2001.
http://www.ncbi.nlm.nih.gov/pubmed/11459730

214. Pollycove, M. & Feinendegen, L. E. Radiation-induced versus endogenous DNA damage: possible effect of inducible protective responses in mitigating endogenous damage. *Hum Exp Toxicol* **22**, 290-306, 2003.
http://www.ncbi.nlm.nih.gov/pubmed/12856953

215. Gasser, S. & Raulet, D. H. The DNA damage response arouses the immune system. *Cancer Res* **66**, 3959-3962, 2006.
http://www.ncbi.nlm.nih.gov/pubmed/16618710

216. Farooque, A. *et al.* Low-dose radiation therapy of cancer: role of immune enhancement. *Expert Rev Anticancer Ther* **11**, 791-802, 2011.
http://www.ncbi.nlm.nih.gov/pubmed/21554054

217. Hall, E. J. & Giaccia, A. J. *Radiobiology for the radiologist*. 6th edn, (Lippincott Williams & Wilkins, 2006). https://lccn.loc.gov/2005031128

ABOUT THE AUTHOR

Mohan Doss has a PhD in Physics and has certification as a Member of Canadian College of Physicists in Medicine in the field of Nuclear Medicine Physics. He works as a medical physicist providing physics support for diagnostic imaging techniques which involve the exposure of patients to ionizing radiation.

Dr. Doss began a detailed study of the health effects of low-level radiation to investigate the claims of publications that there is increased cancer risk in patients due to the radiation exposure from CT scans. His study of the scientific literature revealed that the claims had no merit and that the radiation exposure corresponding to a few CT scans could reduce cancer risk.

As he studied the subject further, he came to realize the very important role the immune system plays in preventing cancers. This led him to propose the concept that cancer may be prevented and treated by boosting the immune system with multiple interventions. This is a very good approach for dealing with cancer as the interventions have very few adverse side effects, and have already shown significant cancer preventive and therapeutic effects. Of course, considerable amount of research including clinical trials are needed to validate and optimize the suggested approach. He has written this book to share the information regarding this approach with the public and the professionals. He welcomes feedback from the readers regarding the book via the book website: https://bit.ly/2E1JHxj or e-mail: i4r@mail.com.

Dr. Doss has over 80 publications in peer-reviewed journals. He is one of the founding members of the group Scientists for Accurate Radiation Information (SARI) and the founder-president of the XLNT Foundation. He is the recipient of the 2014 Outstanding Leadership Award in the Field of Dose-Response presented by the International Dose-Response Society. He lives in Philadelphia, PA with his wife Padma.

Disclaimer: Please note that the views presented in this book are the author's professional opinions and do not necessarily represent the views of his employer or the organizations he is affiliated with.